GOOD PRACTICE IN CHILD PROTECTION

Christine Hobart ● **Jill Frankel**

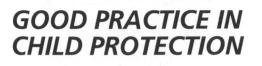

First published in 1998 by:
Stanley Thornes (Publishers) Ltd

Reprinted in 2001 by:
Nelson Thornes Ltd
Delta Place
27 Bath Road
CHELTENHAM
GL53 7TH
United Kingdom

02 03 04 05 06 / 13 12 11 10 9 8 7 6 5

A catalogue record for this book is available from the British Library

ISBN 0 7487 3094 X

Page make-up by Columns Design Ltd

Printed and bound in Spain by GraphyCems

CONTENTS

ABOUT THE AUTHORS

Christine Hobart, Cert Ed., RHV, RGN, FWT, was Curriculum Area Manager at City and Islington College. She was an external and internal examiner for CACHE, and is a child-care assessor for NVQs. She retired from teaching in 1997, to concentrate on writing and on consultancy work.

Jill Frankel, MA Child Development, B.Ed., was Course Tutor at the same college. She has been an internal examiner for CACHE.

The authors come from a background of health visiting and nursery education, and worked together in Camden before meeting again at City and Islington College. For nine years they were part of a course team, involved in the development of many innovative courses for CACHE, including the Camden Training Centre Course for Unemployed Adults, the Orthodox Jewish Certificate in Child-care for the Hassedic community, the three year part-time Diploma Course, and the Certificate in Playskills.

This book is the fifth one, published by Stanley Thornes, by the authors writing together. In some ways it has been the most difficult to write, but also the most worthwhile.

DEDICATIONS

We dedicate this book to Jordan, Richard, Katie, Jamie, Miles, Jason, Lisa and Charlie.

ACKNOWLEDGEMENTS

We would like to thank our colleagues at City and Islington College for their support and encouragement.

We are particularly indebted to Angela Dare whose clear thinking, knowledge and common sense was, as ever, generously provided.

A special thank you also to Pat Loizou and Liza Martello for reading and commenting on some of the issues.

This book could not have been written without the children and families with whom we have worked and the students we have taught and from whom we have learnt so much.

The outline procedure for investigating a case of possible child abuse on page 35 (from *Child Protection in Early Childhood Services* [1994]); and the principles set out on pages 23–4 (from *A Policy for Young Children* [1990]), are reproduced by kind permission of the National Children's Bureau. 'Anti-discriminatory Practice' on pages 28–9 (© London Borough of Islington) is reproduced by kind permission of Islington Area Child Protection Committee. The child protection process on page 33 is adapted from *Child Protection: A Guide for Midwives* by Jenny Fraser, published by Books for Midwives, 174a Ashley Road, Hale, Cheshire WA15 9SF. The day nursery start form on pages 49–50 is reproduced by kind permission of the University of London Union. 'The extent of violence involving children' on page 59, from 'Children and Violence: the Report of the Commission on Children and Violence' convened by the Gulbenkian Foundation, is reproduced by kind permission of the Calouste Gulbenkian Foundation. 'Child Protection Policy' on page 81 is reproduced by kind permission of Susan Hay, Nursery Works. 'What Places Children at Risk of Child Abuse?' on page 115 is reproduced from *Child Abuse and Neglect: An Introduction, Workbook 1 Making Sense of Child Abuse* by kind permission of the Open University.

The authors and publishers have made every effort to trace the owners of copyright material. Should copyright have been unwittingly infringed in this book, the owners should contact the publishers who will make corrections at reprint.

THE NEEDS OF CHILDREN

The needs of children are defined by Alice Miller in her book *The Drama of Being a Child*, published by Virago Press, 1988.

1 'All children are born to grow, to develop, to live, to love, and to articulate their needs and feelings for their self protection.

2 'For their development children need the respect and protection of adults who take them seriously, love them, and honestly help them to become orientated in the world.

3 'When these vital needs are frustrated and children are instead abused for the sake of adults' needs by being exploited, beaten, punished, taken advantage of, manipulated, neglected, or deceived without the intervention of any witness, then their integrity will be lastingly impaired.'

INTRODUCTION

Since the authors first worked together in a London Borough in 1976, as a Health Visitor and a Nursery Teacher in an inner London school, society has developed a much greater understanding of the complex problems of child abuse and neglect. We have a much clearer view of what we can do to protect children and to work with children and families in partnership.

We have become aware that children of any age, sex, race, religion and socioeconomic background can become victims of abuse and neglect. We now know that large numbers of children at risk are never reported to agencies who can help them and their families and, indeed, that many children thought to be at risk have not been helped. In May 1997, doubt was cast about the large numbers of children returned to their families following the Cleveland affair. It is clear that no one professional or agency can work alone; everyone in the community must work together to effectively identify and prevent child abuse and neglect, and provide help, support and therapy for those children who have become victims and for the families involved.

This book is especially written for child-care practitioners who are in the forefront when the abuse of young children is disclosed and are often expected to support and help the families and the children, with very little guidance. We are aware of the stress and distress caused by caring for children who have been abused or neglected and a good sound knowledge of procedures, guidelines and good practice should go some way to alleviating these feelings.

1 THE HISTORY OF CHILD ABUSE

It is by looking at the history of childhood that we make our judgements about child abuse today. History is used as a means of casting light on present issues. Some people feel that whatever is happening today is an improvement on the past, while others look at past centuries through rose-coloured spectacles.

We have no concrete evidence of how children were treated in earlier times. We take our ideas from contemporary paintings and literature. There were few child-care manuals, and no films or photographs to back up theories of child-rearing practices.

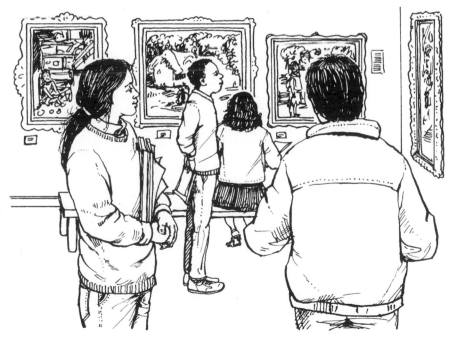

Paintings may provide a clue as to how children were treated in the past

Historical perspectives

All historical writing is inevitably selective, and different historians have very different ideas about the concept of childhood up to the nineteenth century.

In the early part of the last century, child mortality rates were so high that it has been suggested that parents were obliged to limit the amount of emotional involvement with their young children, although this is impossible to prove. Large families were the norm, as infant mortality claimed between 50 and 75 per cent of children before the age of 5. It was not until the mid-nineteenth century that infant mortality rates decreased, thanks to better awareness of public health and sanitation.

Infant mortality rates (deaths of infants under one year of age, per thousand live births) in the UK:	
1900–02	142
1910–12	110
1920–22	82
1930–32	67
1950–52	30
1960–62	22
1970–72	18
1980–82	12
1990–92	7
1990	7.9
1991	7.4
1992	6.6
1993	6.3
1994	6.2
1995	6.2

From 1900 to 1902 the number of 1- to 4-year-olds who died was 62,725. In 1995, in the same age group, 735 children died.

Activity
Visit the oldest part of your local cemetery and see how many tombstones refer to children under the age of 8. Is the cause of death mentioned?

What seems sure is that, until the last century, children were not seen as independent citizens, but as the property of their parents. This still holds true in some countries where children may be maimed by their parents to earn money by begging, or made to work from a very young age. China's policy of restricting family size to one child in urban areas has possibly led to the abandonment of girl children.

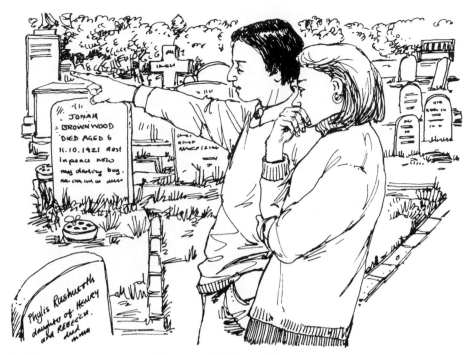

A visit to a cemetery provides an insight into infant mortality

To think about

Now that it is possible to know the sex of a child before birth, should abortion of an unwanted foetus be allowed so that a child brought to term would be of the preferred gender? Do you think that this would reduce the incidence of child abuse?

One can read many accounts of cruelty experienced during childhood written over the centuries. There are naturally more accounts by well-educated people as they would be more likely to write their experiences down, but that does not mean to say that abuse did not take place throughout society. Literature often throws up evidence of child abuse and infanticide. Charles Dickens illustrates in many of his books the plight of abused and neglected children in the last century. You have only to read *Oliver Twist* or *David Copperfield* to understand what many young children endured. Charles Kingsley's *The Water Babies* describes the life of small children forced to sweep chimneys. More recently, the books of Jeannette Winterson, Maya Angelou and others describe the horrors of an unprotected childhood. Celebrities such as Oprah Winfrey and Roseanne Barr have been open about the abuse they suffered as children and this may have encouraged other survivors to speak out and to come to terms with their feelings.

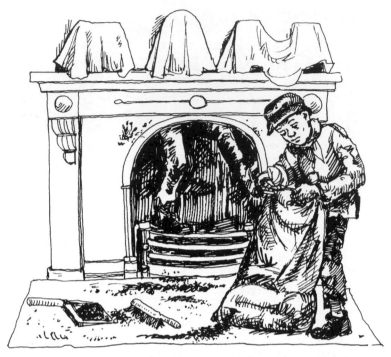

As recently as the 19th century young children were forced to sweep chimneys

Activity
Suggest two books, either autobiographical or fictional, written within the last twenty years, in which the authors describe an unhappy childhood caused by abuse or neglect.

From what we read, it seems that the distinction between children and adults was not so clear cut as it is today. In the Middle Ages the concept of childhood did not seem to exist and once children had become physically competent between the ages of 5 and 8 years old, they became part of the adult community and were expected to earn their keep. By the beginning of the nineteenth century concern was being expressed and the needs of children were being shown in books discussing child rearing. Legislation recognising children's needs and rights was made distinct from that of adults and by 1952 it became possible to bring care proceedings without first prosecuting the parents. You will find all the relevant Acts protecting children at the end of the book in Appendix 1.

In 1946 Caffey, a radiologist, published a paper describing patterns of multiple fractures and subdural haematoma in small children. He speculated that they could be the result of injury rather than disease. In 1953 Silverman suggested that injuries might result from parental neglect but referred to the notion of 'accident proneness'. In 1955 Woolley and Evans suggested the possibility of injury caused deliberately by parents or caregivers.

The sixties onwards

The breakthrough in public awareness concerning non-accidental injury came towards the end of the sixties, and was the result of work presented by Dr Henry Kempe and his colleagues in Denver, Colorado in the USA. He was a paediatrician and his paper published in 1962 was *The Battered Child Syndrome.* This emotive term ensured public attention. In the UK, two orthopaedic surgeons, Griffiths and Moynihan, coined the term 'battered baby'. In 1966 the British Paediatric Association published guidance to members about the management of these cases. In 1965 Professor Keith Simpson of the Department of Forensic medicine at the University of London published a paper referring to a father recently convicted of the murder of two of his children. Arguing that both infants were typical of the 'battered baby' syndrome, he suggested that GPs should take on the role of investigator in such cases. Dr Camps, another forensic scientist, at the London Hospital, argued that the incidence of this syndrome was widespread, and called for the full co-operation of the medical, legal and social authorities. Up until this point it was mainly the medical profession in the UK who were highlighting the issues, and many of their recommendations concerned GPs and casualty house officers, insisting that they became more aware of the children at risk. Awareness outside the medical profession was very limited and members of the legal and social welfare agencies were not involved centrally. The emphasis of social work was still to keep families together and to prevent delinquency.

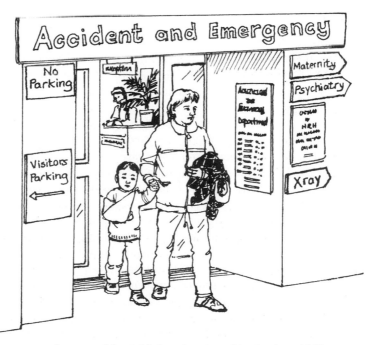

Public awareness of non-accidental injury increased in the late 1960s

In 1968 the NSPCC Battered Child Research Unit was established, publishing many papers between 1969 and 1977. It was this unit that took on the role of educating other professional groups and ensured that the issue was taken up by the media and the government and eventually led to the establishment of special units. A paediatrician, Professor John Davis, the Chair of the Manchester Child Abuse Policy Committee invited the submission of proposals 'to provide a specialist service. This was to help the community services, both statutory and voluntary, deal adequately with families who severely maltreat their children, as is seen in the clinical conditions known as 'the battered child syndrome'. The NSPCC unit would be available for consultation and case work service where a child under the age of 4 was suspected of receiving injuries other than by accident'. The first unit opened in 1972. The age range was later extended from 4 to 16.

During the sixties and seventies the emphasis was less on cruelty and punishment and more on preventative and therapeutic action. The trend was to keep families together at almost all costs and it was assumed that parents who battered must have had terrible childhoods themselves. To some extent there was a polarisation of different perspectives between social services and the police in their approach.

To think about
How might differences in approach militate against these two agencies working together?

In 1970 the NSPCC issued a report suggesting that the increase in publicity and professional education had led to a growth in awareness for the need for intervention in the less obvious cases of abuse. It also stressed the importance of a multi-disciplinary approach and recommended the establishment of central registers of children suspected of being at risk from abuse at local level. The main function would be the identification of repeated abuse within a family and to provide therapy.

There were many terrible cases of children who died of abuse and neglect, but that of Maria Colwell (born 25.3.65, died 7.1.73) who was battered to death by her stepfather after returning from foster care was crucial in establishing the issue as a major social problem, and resulted in fundamental changes in policy and practice.

The publicity given to the brutal killing of this child led to a change in the role of the social worker who would now take on this child protection work as the highest priority. It generated considerable concern and fear, and there was disquiet voiced in the media about the growth, role and activities of social workers. The enquiry into the death of Maria highlighted four main areas of concern:

■ errors of judgement resulting from inexperience and lack of specialist knowledge for those professionally concerned with Maria's welfare
■ communication failures between the agencies, and the need to define roles and ensure they did not overlap
■ social workers have a responsibility to seek out information, but others have a responsibility not to withhold information about children at risk

- inaccuracies and deficiencies in the recording of visits and telephone messages. Dates and times of visits must be recorded, a distinction should be made between fact and impression and the source of all information should be made clear.

CHANGES IN PROCEDURES

At the beginning of the seventies, various DHSS circulars were issued advising the establishment of Area Review Committees (ARCs), including senior representatives of all statutory and voluntary agencies. Among the terms of reference it was suggested that:

- the duties and responsibilities of all people involved with any aspect of non-accidental injury cases should be defined
- local practice and procedures should be devised
- education and training should be provided for all professional people involved
- public awareness should be increased
- procedures should be established to ensure that children did not slip through the net if the family moved to another area

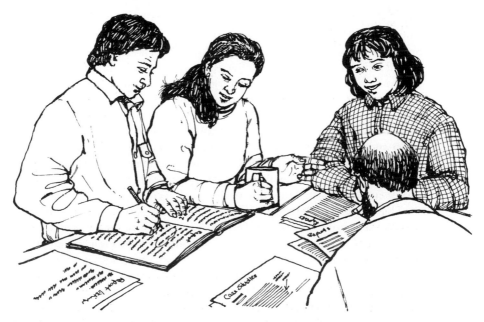

In the 1970s new procedures were set up for dealing with suspected cases of abuse

In 1976, the DHSS advised that all areas should hold a central register of children at risk of abuse and advised on the information that should be recorded. The importance of case conferences (now called child protection conferences) and the need to appoint a key worker to the case was stressed. Later in the year, another circular advised that the police should attend all initial conferences. This multi-disciplinary approach was consolidated in 1980 and extended the criteria for inclusion on the register from physical abuse to severe and persistent neglect and emotional abuse. Sexual abuse was not included unless associated with physical injury.

To think about
Why do you think it took so long for sexual abuse to become an issue for child protection agencies?

Circulars continued to be issued in the 1980s, emphasising the importance of a multi-disciplinary response, and stressing the central social worker with statutory powers in the management and co-ordination of each case. Child abuse registers were re-titled child protection registers. It was recommended that child abuse consultants or advisers should be appointed in every local authority. It was also recommended that sexual abuse should be included in the child abuse framework for the first time.

HELPLINES

The NSPCC have offered confidential help on the telephone for many years. This has been used mainly by adults reporting concerns. In 1986, Childline was established. This was initiated by Esther Rantzen, who felt sure that there were many children suffering from abuse of various types who were unable to speak face to face to adult carers and would value speaking by telephone to an invisible counsellor. She has been vindicated as there have been approximately twenty thousand calls for help every year from physically and sexually abused children. Another 1,300 spoke of fear, neglect or threats made to them. While the majority of calls are about family problems, bullying, pregnancy, drug abuse or running away, one child in four is in danger from assault in some form, according to Childline. A recent survey indicated that one in three callers were unable to make contact.

The role of Childline is to empower children to seek help for themselves, and the counsellors do not generally give direct advice. If they feel a child is in especial danger, they might get in touch with the police in the child's area, but only with the permission of the child.

To think about
It has been said that in spite of current concern about abused children, there has never been a better time to be a child. Do you agree?

During the 1980s there was a number of highly publicised deaths, and social workers were often held to blame when events went tragically wrong in failing to protect children. In 1987, in Cleveland, a large number of children, in a short period of time, were removed from their parents following allegations of sexual abuse. The allegations were substantiated by a rather controversial medical test. In

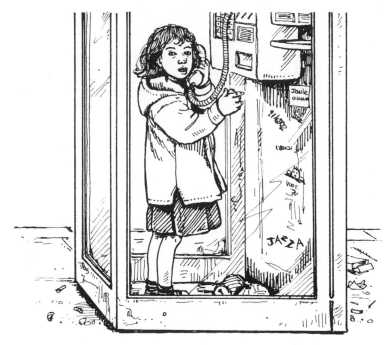

Childline enables a child to speak to a counsellor by telephone

1987, between March and July, 104 children were removed from their homes. Many of these children were later thought to have been removed unnecessarily, and doctors and social workers were blamed for being over zealous. In 1997, a three part television documentary, *The Death of Childhood*, appeared to suggest that many of the children who were returned home had, in fact, been abused.

THE CHILDREN ACT, 1989

By the end of the eighties there was concern over the conflicting areas of family privacy, the accountability of professional power and the rights of children. The Children Act, 1989, was drawn up to address these areas, and to make the law simpler and easier to use. The Act contains three major principles:
- the welfare of the child is paramount
- there should be as little delay as possible by the court in deciding issues
- the court has to be satisfied that it is better to make an order than not to do so.

The Act also introduces a 'welfare checklist' that the court has a duty to consider in any proceedings, and allows the court to have greater flexibility in its decision-making powers. This would take into account:
- the wishes and feelings of the child subject to the child's age and understanding
- the child's physical, emotional and educational needs
- the likely effect on the child of any change in circumstances

- the age, gender, background and relevant characteristics of the child
- the parents' ability to meet the child's needs
- any harm the child has suffered or is at risk of suffering
- the court's powers under the Children Act.

Up until the mid-sixties, the family appeared to be a secure unit, and the idealised nuclear family was seen as the pivot of values and social mores. The shock of the battered baby syndrome, the death of Maria Colwell and the Cleveland affair have resulted in radical re-thinking about how we perceive and support children and families who are at risk.

Activity
You will probably have in your family people who will remember the death of Maria Colwell. Did they feel shocked at the time? Who did they blame, and do they think it could happen today?

Child abuse inquiries

There are three main types of inquiry:
- an internal inquiry or case review, conducted by senior managers of all concerned agencies
- an external inquiry set up locally, but with an independent chairperson and often with members from outside the area
- a statutory inquiry set up by government.

An inquiry will try to:
- establish the true facts of the case
- determine who was responsible for carrying out certain actions and neglecting others
- look critically at the quality of the work and collaboration of the relevant agencies
- learn from the experience, and recommend changes in legislation, professional responsibilities, and governmental guidelines
- restore confidence in the system, and reassure the general public.

INQUIRIES

As child-care practitioners you may come across, in your reading and training, a number of children whose death from physical abuse or neglect resulted in an inquiry.

Maria Colwell, aged 8 years, was killed by her stepfather in 1973, shortly after being returned home from her foster parents. Neighbours and her school reported evidence of rejection and physical abuse. She was subject to a supervision order at the time of her death.

Susan Auckland was killed by her father in 1974, at the age of 15 months. At the end of the trial it was stated that he had also killed his nine-week-old daughter,

Marianne, in 1968. The father was sentenced to five years imprisonment for manslaughter.

Jasmine Beckford, aged $4\frac{1}{2}$ years, was killed by her stepfather in July 1984. She was neglected and abused over a long period by both parents. Jasmine had attended a nursery but had very poor attendance. She was withdrawn from the nursery ten months before her death. She was in the care of the local authority when she was killed.

Tyra Henry was killed by her father in September, 1984, when she was 22 months, while still legally in the care of the local authority. Her mother became pregnant with Tyra's brother Tyrone, at the age of 15. The father assaulted Tyrone when he was 4 months old, leaving him blind and brain damaged, and he was removed into long-term care. The father was convicted of cruelty and subsequent to this a care order was made on Tyra when she was born, and she remained on this at the time of her death.

Kimberley Carlile, aged $4\frac{1}{2}$ years, was killed by her stepfather in 1986. She had been tortured and starved for many weeks before her death. There were concerns while the family was living in the Wirral. When they moved to Greenwich, Social Services attempted to monitor the family, but found it difficult to gain access.

Heidi Koseda died due to the neglect of her mother and her mother's partner in 1985. She had been well cared for until her parents separated when she was 2, and her mother began to live with a man known for his violent behaviour. Neighbours had complained to the NSPCC that Heidi had not been seen. Heidi was locked away in a room and died of starvation. It was two months before her body was found.

Rikki Neave, aged 6 years, was found dead in 1994. His mother was cleared of his murder, but given seven years imprisonment for cruelty. The inquiry is to be carried out in 1997 by social services inspectors.

Activity
Research into one of these distressing cases, and report your findings back to your college group. Ensure you cover the following areas.
1 What agencies were involved in the case? Comment on how well they worked together.
2 What signs of concern were evident before the child's death?
3 Had the child's health and developmental progress been monitored?
4 Were there any important cultural factors? Were there any signs of stereotyping?
5 Did the case change future practice and legislation?

Child sexual abuse

Until the 1980s, the realisation that young children from birth onwards could be sexually abused had not been recognised by the general public or by most professionals. In 1986 Childline was established and for the first time, the public was made aware that very young children were disclosing sexual abuse in very large numbers.

In 1987 two doctors, Hobbs and Wynne, published an influential paper presenting evidence that boys as well as girls were sexually abused, and that very small children, even babies might be victims of such abuse. It was also apparent that it occurred in all sections of society. In the same year, a newspaper reported that a large number of angry parents had their children removed from their care on the basis of a medical diagnosis carried out by two consultant paediatricians. The procedures were not in place to cope with the

- conflicting medical opinions
- spiralling referrals from different agencies
- conflict over the correct method of examination
- extent and nature of parental involvement
- failure of communication
- over-full hospital wards
- distraught parents and upset children.

An inquiry was set up, and the recommendations that followed were summarised by the briefing from the Children's Legal Centre on page 13.

The fact that a child does not die from sexual abuse means that, although the perpetrator may be brought to court, there is rarely a local or an official inquiry. It is only when there are a number of children involved as in the Cleveland inquiry (121 children), or in organised abuse (sometimes referred to as Satanic or ritual abuse) as in Nottingham (1988, 23 children), Rochdale (1991, 20 children), Manchester (1991, 13 children) and the Orkney Islands (1991, 9 children) that the media becomes involved, and public awareness is aroused. There have been a number of inquiries into abuse in residential homes, again involving large numbers of children.

To think about

In any community, where there are large numbers of children said to be sexually abused, what impact would this have on a local nursery? What would be the role of the child-care practitioner?

Current times

THE INFLUENCE OF THE MEDIA

The media includes:

- newspapers, books and magazines
- television and radio
- theatre, cinema and video
- computers and the Internet.

Newspapers have always played a role in keeping the general public informed and educated about child protection issues. In 1996 and 1997 investigative journalism

Children's Legal Centre Briefing
THE CLEVELAND INQUIRY REPORT'S RECOMMENDATIONS ON CHILDREN

'There is a danger that in looking to the welfare of the children believed to be the victims of sexual abuse the children themselves may be overlooked. The child is a person and not an object of concern.

'We recommend that:

a   Professionals recognise the need for adults to explain to children what is going on. Children are entitled to a proper explanation appropriate to their age, to be told why they are being taken away from home and given some idea of what is going to happen to them.

b   Professionals should not make promises which cannot be kept to a child, and in the light of possible court procedings should not promise a child that what is said in confidence can be kept in confidence.

c   Professionals should always listen carefully to what the child has to say and take seriously what is said.

d   Throughout the proceedings the views and the wishes of the child particularly as to what should happen to him/her, should be taken into consideration by the professionals involved with their problems.

e   The views and wishes of the child should be placed before whichever court deals with the case. We do not, however, suggest that those wishes should predominate.

f   Children should not be subjected to repeated medical examinations solely for evidential purposes. Where appropriate, according to age and understanding, the consent of the child should be obtained before any medical examination or photography.

g   Children should not be subjected to repeated interviews nor to the probing and confrontational type of 'disclosure' interview for the same purpose, for it in itself can be damaging and harmful to them. The consent of the child should where possible be obtained before the interviews are recorded on video.

h   The child should be medically examined and interviewed in a suitable and sensitive environment, where there are suitably trained staff available.

I   When a child is moved from home or between hospital and foster home it is important that those responsible for the day to day care of the child not only understand the child's legal status but also have sufficient information to look after the child properly.

j   Those involved in investigation of child sexual abuse should make a conscious effort to ensure that they act throughout in the best interests of the child'.

Report of the Inquiry into Child Abuse in Cleveland 1987

unveiled rampant abuse in children's residential homes in Merseyside and in Wales. Many of the children who were abused in the past committed suicide, while others have found their lives ruined. The publicity has led to government action to tighten standards in children's homes.

Journalists become interested in child abuse matters when the numbers of children abused are very large, or the perpetrator is someone well-known, or the abuse of an individual child results in death. It was the media's attention to the death of Maria Colwell that focused the general public's attention, and pushed forward changes in practice.

Journalists sometimes seem to enjoy pointing out the failure of authorities and social workers and the reporting itself is often one-sided. Nevertheless, the media has contributed a great deal to the progress made over the last quarter of a century to ensure that the systems for protecting children now in place are more effective. Keeping the balance between the right to privacy and the public's right to know is a difficult task. Preserving confidentiality in the traditional sense can contribute to the preservation of the family 'secret'. The recent use of surveillance video cameras in hospital paediatric wards has revealed instances of abuse by parents.

Activity
Read a range of newspapers over a period of a month. Collect all the articles and reports on child abuse. Compare the different viewpoints of the broadsheets (such as the *Guardian*) and the tabloids (such as the *Daily Mirror*).

Television, plays and films often draw large audiences when depicting an episode of child abuse. Abusers are sometimes shown in a sympathetic light, and the general public may gain some understanding of the factors which lead to abuse. The televising of the Louise Woodward case alerted the public and, possibly due to the sympathy aroused, her conviction for murder was changed to manslaughter and her sentence reduced.

Pornographic videos which are carelessly left around or deliberately shown to children, expose children to films which may show sex in a sadistic or bestial way, and may disturb children and have a negative influence on their behaviour.

THE INTERNET

The Internet is used by over fifty million people world-wide, and offers widening horizons and new educational opportunities to children and their families. Unfortunately, it has also given paedophiles access to each other, and some of the messages relayed are most disturbing, presenting images of children engaged in sexual activity, and has allowed paedophiles to present themselves as children in order to make contact. The Internet also makes pornography easily available and this seems to be happening to children at an earlier and earlier age. There is much debate about the need to exercise more control over the content of images on the Internet, and it is hoped legislation will shortly be in place to deal with this problem. A recent warning by the National Children Homes Action for Children stated that children can stumble accidentally on pictures of explicit material. A software company has developed a programme, Safety-Net, which identifies and prevents specified types of pictures and words or access to certain Internet groups. There are government proposals in the UK to censor access to the Internet.

THE DANGERS OF RESIDENTIAL CARE

When children have been abused and the courts decide that they need a place of safety, they may be placed in residential care. This is not always such a safe place.

In December 1996, the *Independent* reported that police had launched a full scale investigation into allegations of sexual and physical abuse in children's homes in Merseyside in the north-west of England. Around three thousand children were thought to have been involved in fifteen homes. The allegations of abuse stretched back over twenty years. The abuse was thought to be systematic, involving paedophile activity, with children being moved between homes.

In January 1997, the same newspaper reported on another major abuse inquiry – many hundreds children were alleged to have been sexually abused in children's homes across North Wales, involving many staff and six police officers. The role of the insurers of the councils in North Wales was also to be investigated, as it was further alleged that it was these insurers who caused the council to turn a blind eye to what was going on, as any inquiry would be too expensive.

The £6 million public inquiry, chaired by Sir William Utting, into the case showed that 650 children were physically and sexually abused, and that up to eighty staff were involved. Social services were criticised for being, at the very least, careless as to the plight of many children in their care, or at worst, negligent to the point of gross professional incompetence, or even guilty of 'closing their eyes'. The findings were published in November 1997, urging the government to regulate private foster care, bring small homes into line with larger ones, set up a specialist group to develop a child-care strategy for residential care, and be more vigilant in checking the backgrounds of potential employees.

A similar scandal in Cheshire is thought to involve more than four thousand children, and in Clwyd six care workers were jailed for offences against children.

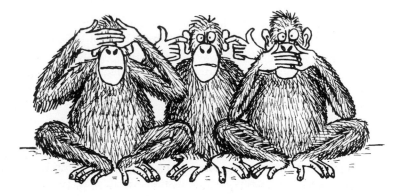

Very many cases of abuse go unreported

Other types of abuse have been reported. 'Pin down', where children are confined to their rooms for long periods without any contact with other people, has been recommended in the past for unruly children. This punishment has now been shown to be cruel.

It would appear that unless abuse involves very large numbers of children, very little gets reported or brought to the notice of the public.

There are obviously many well run homes that do a good job. Most of the children who live in residential homes have experienced trauma and emotional deprivation in their own families, and they deserve the quality of care enjoyed by most children in supportive families. They must be protected from further abuse.

One of the problems is that, despite requirements for disclosure of criminal background and police checks, some sex offenders are clever and persuasive enough to gain employment time and again with young and vulnerable children.

To think about

Is it safer to leave some abused children at home, as the risk of putting them into residential care might be greater? What would be the best care for some of these children?

Many local authorities now prefer to place children with foster carers, rather than in residential care, but this too has its dangers, both for the child and the family. The foster carers need to be selected and vetted very carefully, and will require training and support. Older foster children in the family, who have been abused themselves, have been known to abuse younger children in the foster family. Not all foster parents have the emotional resources themselves to cope with very disturbed unhappy children.

Global issues

EMPLOYMENT IN OTHER COUNTRIES

UNICEF recently reported that some 250 million children are having to work in dangerous, unacceptable conditions, mostly in Asia, Africa and Latin America. The true figure could be much higher as most of the work is both unseen and unreported. In some countries, the high incidence of HIV and AIDS has left many children orphaned. The report describes many of the risks including:

- inhaling pesticides
- undertaking heavy manual labouring
- exposure to snake and insect bites.

The report calls for free compulsory primary education in developing countries.

Some of the goods sold in the UK are made by children held in virtual slavery in factories abroad. A report by Christian Aid in May 1997 has highlighted the scandal of young children in India employed in making sports goods for export, often being paid as little as 12p a day. The International Labour Organisation

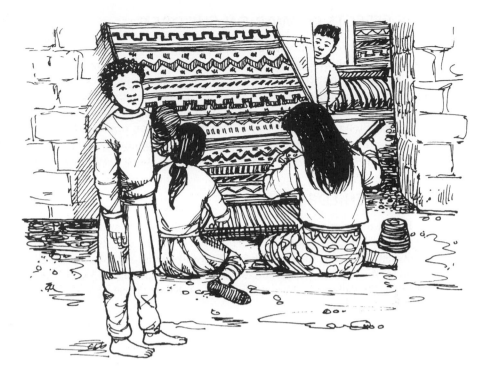

In some countries children work in poor conditions in factories for slave wages

(ILO) faces the gigantic task of organising governments, employers and Trade Unions to secure agreements of industry-wide standards that prevent exploitation of children and 'ban other employment practices which are incompatible with human rights and labour standards'.

CHILD ACTORS AND MODELS

Although most children who model or act are well protected, both by a sensible family and by the agencies, there have been cases where children are exploited in an explicitly sexual way. In the USA, there are competitions held for very young children, from the age of 3, who are trained to perform for an adult audience in a pseudo-mature way. The competitions are held all over the country. In a recent case, one of these children was raped and murdered in very suspicious circumstances and the murderer has still not been charged. Even if no significant harm comes to such children, at the very least they lose a valuable part of their childhood. It is alleged that Michael Jackson, who was made to work from the age of 5 years, now compensates for his lost childhood by having a theme park as part of his home and seeking the company of children

THE EFFECTS OF WAR ON CHILDREN

Many regimes conscript young children into the army – the recent war in Rwanda enlisted many thousands of such children. Although the war appears to be over, the damaging after-effects can last for decades. Some countries use systematic forced conscription of children. UNICEF recently stated that 2 million children have been killed in global wars in the past decade, and the situation is worsening. Up to 5 million children have been disabled, 1 million orphaned or separated from parents, and some 10 million psychologically traumatised by war. Most children who die are not killed by bombs or bullets but succumb to starvation or sickness.

STREET CHILDREN

In Brazil, many abandoned children live on the streets and the rubbish dumps. It has been alleged that police frequently 'clean up' the streets by murdering as many of these children as they can find. We should not be complacent about street children in the UK, as many runaways congregate in big cities and are at risk of exploitation, pornography, prostitution and drug trafficking.

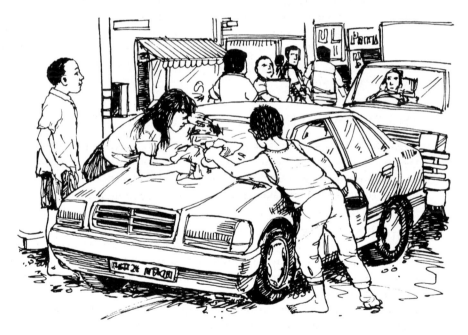

Many runaway children end up living on the streets

Activity
There are other forms of exploitation. Research the sale, trafficking and abduction of children. Find out about the use of children in medical research.

SEX TOURISM

UNICEF recently stated that an estimated one million children world-wide are reportedly forced into the sex market annually. The first world congress against the commercial sexual exploitation of children was held in Sweden in 1996. In the UK it became law in July 1996 to force UK citizens and residents to be tried in the UK for offences committed against children abroad. There are several countries notorious for exploiting children for sex, particularly Thailand, the Philippines and Sri Lanka and an expanding tourist industry has seen the growth in tourists travelling to these countries for sexual gratification with young children. These activities have seen an increase in the incidence of HIV and AIDS, and in the numbers of children being born who do not receive financial support from their fathers.

Save the Children recently warned of a world-wide expansion of the child sex industry and of the global sexual exploitation of children by paedophiles. Increasing numbers of children are becoming involved, not only in prostitution but also in child trafficking and pornography. Poverty is identified as a critical factor in the growth of the child sex industry. This is a global issue and happens in Britain as well as in many other countries. Save the Children recently produced a report, *Kids for Hire*.

THE RECOVERED/FALSE MEMORY DEBATE

Frederick Crew described recovered memory in an influential two-part article in the *New York Review of Books*: 'A single diagnosis for miscellaneous complaints – that of unconsciously repressed sexual abuse in childhood – has grown, in the past decade, from virtual non-existence to epidemic frequency. The comment has been made that this may be of considerable commercial value to some psychiatrists and therapists across America'.

There is nothing new in the recovered memory theory, as it is similar to the one that Freud proposed over a hundred years ago. He claimed that psychological illness was often caused by sexual abuse which had been forgotten and repressed. What is different is the numbers involved and the fact that any abnormal behaviour indicator is immediately attributed to repressed memories of sexual abuse. The 'victims' are encouraged to confront the alleged perpetrators and as a result many families have been torn apart. No corroboration is asked for and therapists refuse to meet the family as they say it is betrayal of trust in the patient.

This notion has now crossed the Atlantic, and the first case was reported in Britain in 1990. Many of the alleged perpetrators were instrumental in founding The British False Memory Society in 1993, which has more than 400 cases on its books (the US equivalent has 12,000). Recently the British Psychological Society

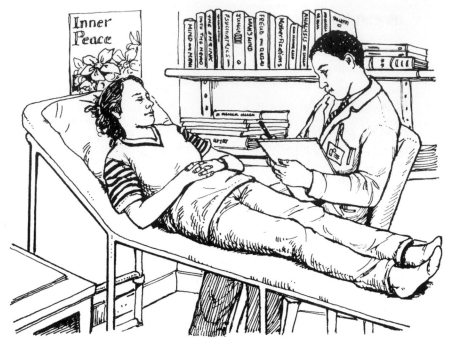

The 1990s have seen a huge increase in the instances of recovered memory

pronounced that both true and false memories can be recovered but that it is very hard to distinguish between them without additional evidence or corroboration. Both can be convincing. Therapists should convey that uncertainty to the patient.

Allan Levy, QC, stated recently that the topic of false memory syndrome has given rise to more emotion than reason and can throw doubt on genuine child sexual abuse cases.

We have seen in this chapter how infant mortality has been dramatically reduced in this century and how society has responded to distressing cases of child abuse. There are still many issues concerning child protection which need to be addressed. A recent publication, issued by the Department of Health, entitled *Child Protection: Messages from Research*, highlighted the findings of twenty research studies and has identified three main areas of interest.

■ How is abuse defined in the context of normal childhood experience, and how do we estimate the incidence of different types of abuse and neglect in society?

■ How can we achieve the protection and safety of children, and who is involved in this process?

■ How can we establish good practice in all stages of the child protection process?

As a professional child-care practitioner, you will be alert to all issues concerning children and keep up to date in your reading. Practice and procedures used to protect children are constantly being evaluated and reassessed in the light of current research and debate. Children have many needs: love, shelter, stimulation, security and nourishment, but meeting these needs counts for nothing unless children are adequately protected.

Resources

Aries, P., *Centuries of Childhood*, Penguin, 1962

Brazler, C., 'Child labour' in *New Internationalist* magazine, July, 1997

de Mause, Loyd, *The History of Childhood*, Condor Books, Souvenir Press, 1973

HMSO, *Child Abuse: a Study of Inquiry Reports 1980-1989*, 1991; *Child Protection: Messages from Research*, 1995

Kempe, R.S. and Kempe, C.H., *Child Abuse*, Developing Child Series, Fontana, 1978

Reder, P., Duncan, S. and Gray, M., *Beyond Blame*, Routledge, 1993

Reid Dr D.H.S., *Suffer the Little Children (Orkney Child Abuse Scandal)*, Medical Institute for Research in Child Cruelty, 1992

Stead, J., 'Caught in the net' in *Nursery World*: 3.10.96

Wallace, W., Look who's watching' in *Nursery World*: 25.9.97

Woodden, K., *Weeping in the Playtime of Others*, McGraw Hill Paperbacks, 1976

2 THE RIGHTS OF CHILDREN AND THE LEGAL FRAMEWORK

> **This chapter covers:**
> - The rights of children
> - The Children Act, 1989
> - Child protection orders
> - Going to court
> - Local procedures
> - Referrals and investigations
> - The child protection conference
> - The child protection register
> - Reviews and de-registration
> - The registration of child-care practitioners
> - Resources

To play an effective part in protecting children in your care, it is important for you to have a clear understanding of the rights of children, the legal framework, and the national and local guidelines published for all professionals working with children. For a long time common law has required any person looking after a child to protect him or her from physical harm by providing the necessities of life, based on need. Statutory responsibility for child protection rests with the Social Services Department of the local authority.

The rights of children

In November, 1959, the UN issued a document declaring the rights of the child. This was motivated by the parlous plight of some children due to wars and famine: children left without parents, families and homes. The following rights are set out.

1 The right to equality, regardless of race, colour, religion, sex or nationality.
2 The right to healthy mental and physical development.
3 The right to a name and a nationality.
4 The right to sufficient food, housing and medical care.
5 The right to special care, if handicapped.
6 The right to love, understanding and care.
7 The right to free education, play and recreation.
8 The right to medical aid in the event of disasters and emergencies.
9 The right to protection from cruelty, neglect and exploitation.
10 The right to protection from persecution and to an upbringing in the spirit of world-wide brotherhood and peace.

Thirty years later, in 1989, the Convention was adopted and further points were added.

Applicable to child protection was the statement that it is:

■ the right of every child to a standard of living adequate for the child's physical, mental, spiritual, moral and social development.

The Convention contains more than thirty articles incorporating civil, economic, social and cultural rights. Article 3, 'The Welfare Principle' states that:

■ in all actions concerning children, whether undertaken by public or private social welfare institutions, courts of law, administrative authorities or legislative bodies, the best interests of the child shall be a primary consideration.

Article 19 defines Protection from Abuse. It aims:

■ to protect the child from all forms of physical or mental violence, injury or abuse, neglect or negligent treatment, maltreatment or exploitation including sexual abuse while in the care of parent/s, legal guardian/s or any other person who has the care of the child.

Protective measures include:

■ support for the child and identification, reporting, referral, investigation, treatment, and follow-up of instances of child maltreatment.

Article 34 concerns protecting the child from sexual abuse and sexual exploitation. This is defined as:

■ inducement or coercion of a child to engage in any unlawful sexual activity
■ exploitative use of children in prostitution or other unlawful sexual practices
■ exploitative use of children in pornographic performances and materials.

It is clear that in many countries it would be impossible to grant all these rights, as even the basic needs for food and shelter cannot be met. It is an important document, however, in recognising the rights of children who have been abused. We need to understand the rights of children and respect them.

Activity
Identify some countries where it currently would not be possible to implement all children's rights. What factors are usually present?

In 1990 The National Children's Bureau set out their Policy for Young Children, in particular the under-5s. The principles of this policy are:

■ that young children are important in their own right and as a resource for the future
■ that young children are valued and their full development is possible only if they live in an environment which reflects and respects their individual identity, culture and heritage
■ that parents are primarily responsible for nurturing and supporting the development of their children and that this important role should be more highly valued in society
■ that central and local government have a duty, working in partnership with parents, to ensure that services and support are available for families: services that encourage children's cognitive, social, emotional and physical development;

and meet parents' needs for support for themselves and for day care for their children.

■ that services for young children should be provided within a consistent legal framework which allows for flexibility but which ensures basic protection against pain and abuse, equal opportunities and the absence of discrimination, and development of the child as an individual through good quality child-care practice.

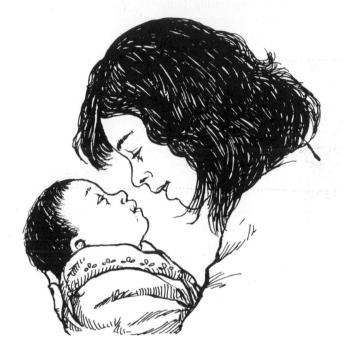

GOOD PRACTICE

Explain to children that they have rights.

1 Teach children that everyone has rights which should not be taken away, such as the right to be safe.
2 Teach children that their bodies belong to them, and no one else.
3 Teach children the right to say 'NO' to any touching they do not like. This needs teaching, as children are generally brought up to be obedient and polite to adults.

The Children Act, 1989

The Children Act, 1989, came into force on 14 October 1991. It has had a major impact on the law relating to children, affecting all children and their families.

Much of the old law was abolished and the emphasis of the new law was that parents should have responsibilities for their children, rather than rights over them. Parental responsibility is defined as the rights, duties, powers, responsibilities and authority that, by law, a parent of a child has in relation to the child and to his or her property.

The Children Act acknowledged the importance of the wishes of the child. Parental rights diminish as the child matures. Parental responsibility is a concept that is important when deciding who is in a position to make decisions about the child, and who should be contacted in any legal proceedings.

Those who can hold parental responsibility are:

- the mother, who always has it, whether married or not. She can only lose it when an adoption or freeing order is made
- the natural father who has it jointly with the natural mother if they are married to each other at the time of the child's birth, or subsequently marry. He, too, can only lose it if an adoption or freeing order is made
- the unmarried father may acquire it by agreement with the mother, or by court order
- the step-parent can acquire it by obtaining a residence order and will lose it if that order ends
- the local authority acquires it when obtaining a care order or emergency protection order and loses it when that order ends
- others, such as grandparents may acquire it by court order and will lose it when the order ends.

Parental responsibility may not be surrendered or transferred. It can be shared with a number of persons and/or the local authority. Each individual having parental responsibility may act alone in exercising it, but not in a way that is incompatible with any court order made under the 1989 Act. The Act sets out a series of principles dictating practice and procedure, both in and out of court.

The key messages of the act are shown on pages 26 to 27.

Section 17 of the Children Act states that it is the duty of every local authority to safeguard and promote the welfare of children within their area who are in need, and attempt to promote the upbringing of such children by their families by providing a range and level of services appropriate to those children's needs.

The anti-discriminatory practice guidelines reproduced on pages 28–9 are an example of part of one local authority's child protection procedures.

THE CHILDREN ACT, 1989

PRINCIPLES OF THE ACT
- Children are generally best looked after within their families.
- Parents and guardians retain parental responsibility and work in partnership with the Local Authority.
- No court order to be made unless better than making no order at all.
- The child's welfare is the court's paramount consideration.
- The Local Authority cannot acquire parental responsibility without a court order.
- Orders available to protect children and avoid unwarranted intervention in family life.

DUTIES AND POWERS
- Identify children in need, safeguard and promote their welfare within their families where consistent.
- Provide a range and level of appropriate services.
- Consult child, parent, those with parental responsibility and others whom the agency considers relevant when making decisions about the child.
- Have regard to child's race, religion, culture and language when making decisions about children being looked after.
- Set up representations and complaints procedure and publish its existence.
- Use orders under Parts IV and V if child is suffering or likely to suffer significant harm.

PRINCIPLES AND PRACTICE GUIDE
- Children, young people and their parents should be considered as individuals with a particular needs and potential.
- A child's age, sex, health, personality, race, culture and life experiences are all relevant to any consideration of needs and vulnerability and have to be taken into account when planning or providing help.
- There are unique advantages for children in experiencing normal family life in their own birth family and every effort should be made to preserve the child's home and family links.
- The development of a working partnership with parents is usually the most effective route to providing supplementary or substitute care for their children.

- The wishes of the children should be taken into account. Children should be consulted and kept informed.
- Decisions made in court should be responsive to the needs of children, promote their welfare and reached without undue delay.
- Where children are placed away from home there must be adequate supervision that ensures highest quality substitute parenting with good standards of care and safety.
- Parents; contact with children should be maintained where ever possible.

EQUALITY ISSUES
- Attitudes towards 'The Family' – the influence of institutional, societal and personal belief and experience on assessment and planning.
- Skills and knowledge available to accurately consult with the child, relatives and others.
- Ability to take into account the factors of race, culture, language and religion.
- Ability to understand the effect of disability on the whole family. Parents should be helped to raise the children themselves.
- Openness to working in partnership; developing a combination of anti-discriminatory policies; commitment to guaranteed resource provision; support to enable staff to work with confidence.

The main points of the Children Act 1989

Activity
There are five main factors cited in the document on pages 28 to 29 which might lead to discrimination.
1 Which of these factors might contribute to families being wrongly suspected of child abuse?
2 How, as child-care practitioners working in a socially deprived area, might you contribute to reducing the stress felt by families?

To think about
Women from cultures where male children are valued should have free access to termination of female foetuses. Discuss this with your group.

ANTI-DISCRIMINATORY PRACTICE

Disability and Sensory Impairment

1.7 There is evidence to suggest that children with disabilities are more vulnerable to abuse than children in general. This is as much a result of the way in which society views disability and arranges services for disabled children as of the disability itself.

1.8 Services which are designed to prevent child abuse should be made available to children with disabilities and sensory impairment. Where child protection concerns are identified, children and families affected by disability must not be discriminated against in service provision. Wherever it is possible services must be adapted to make them fully accessible to children and parents with disabilities or sensory impairment.

Child Protection Work with Minority Ethnic Groups

1.9 Child abuse occurs in all cultural, racial and religious groups.

1.10 Minority ethnic communities in Britain have suffered and continue to suffer racism and discrimination including institutional discrimination from official welfare agencies, the health service and the police. The experience of racism may make families from minority ethnic groups understandably suspicious of the motives and actions of official bodies.

1.11 All agencies have a responsibility to ensure that their services are provided in a way which does not further discriminate and which positively promotes the well being of children from black and minority ethnic groups. This will be done by:

- developing a proper understanding of the child's and family's circumstances and needs in the context of their race, religion, language and culture

- developing services where it is necessary to meet specific racial, religious, linguistic and cultural needs

- making sure that all services are planned and delivered in a way that makes possible the full participation of all children and families

- being aware of the strength of different cultures' approaches to child care

- basing investigation and assessment on objective information, not stereotypes

- making sure that staff at all levels of organisation reflect the ethnic make up of the local community.

Sexuality

1.12 Lesbians and gay men have suffered discrimination and prejudice in the field of child care and child protection. There are common public prejudices about the ability of lesbians and gay men to care for and protect children which are not born out by evidence. In the public mind homosexuality is widely confused with paedophilia.

1.13 Work with lesbians and gay men who are parents or carers will be based on an objective and rational assessment of their capacity – not prejudice or sterotype. Lesbian and gay partners of parents must be included in work wherever they have an active role in the care of children. Young people who are lesbian or gay or uncertain as to their sexual orientation have the same right to protection as other young people.

Gender

1.14 Inequalities between men and women in society impact on child care and child protection. Domestic violence, lack of child care provision and lack of financial independence are of particular importance. It is essential that these are fully considered in undertaking child protection work and that services are delivered in a way which actively combats discrimination against women. Women must be enabled to participate fully and equally in all discussion of child protection concerns and in all child protection services.

Social Deprivation

1.15 Poverty, poor standards of housing, and limited facilities for child care are all factors which limit the development and well being of Islington's children and reduce the quality of parenting. The stresses caused by these factors frequently contribute to the background picture in cases of child abuse.

1.16 The local authority and other agencies with obligation in this arena acknowledge their responsibility to alleviate factors which contribute to child abuse – both in general and in individual cases.

1.17 However the existence of practical and material problems – whatever their cause – does not reduce the prime responsibility to focus on the needs and well being of the individual child at all times.

Example of a local authority's anti-discriminatory practice

The Act requires local authorities to set up Area Child Protection Committees (ACPCs) consisting of professionals representing all the agencies involved in caring for children, such as social services, education, police, probation services, health services and voluntary organisations. The ACPCs will:

- establish, maintain and review child protection guidelines and procedures
- monitor the implementation of local procedures
- identify important issues from the management of cases and inquiry reports and implement recommendations
- monitor work on prevention of abuse, and make recommendations
- monitor work on providing treatment and advice
- monitor inter-agency liaison and training, and make recommendations
- conduct case reviews
- publish an annual report.

Activity
Obtain a copy of the Children Act , 1989 or *An Introduction to the Children Act (1989)* published by the Stationery Office, which is easier to read. Make a note of all the sections which refer primarily to child protection.

Child protection orders

Since the implementation of The Children Act, many children at risk of harm can be satisfactorily protected without going to the courts. Where this is not possible, the Act has introduced new Child Protection Orders.

A CHILD ASSESSMENT ORDER

This may be applied for only in court, on notice by a local authority or the NSPCC. It is used when there is reasonable cause to believe that a child is suffering or is likely to suffer significant harm and it would be very difficult to obtain a satisfactory assessment of the child's health and development without such an order. The order lasts for a maximum of seven days.

AN EMERGENCY PROTECTION ORDER

This is intended for use only in real emergencies and enables a child to be made safe, when he or she might otherwise suffer harm. The order lasts for a maximum of eight days and can be extended once only for a further seven days. Anyone can apply to the court for this emergency order. During the time it is in force the local authority will have limited parental responsibility. It may set out who may be allowed or refused contact with the child. It may involve assessment of the child.

A RECOVERY ORDER

If a child who is in care following an emergency protection order or in police protection, is missing, has been abducted or has run away from the person responsible for his or her care, the court may make a recovery order and this will be implemented by the police.

A SUPERVISION ORDER

This will be applied for by the local authority if the authority was unable to make satisfactory voluntary arrangements with the parents to ensure the child's protection. The child is placed under the supervision of the local authority which does not have parental responsibility but does have rights of access to the child to ensure the child's well-being. The order can last up to one year and can be extended.

A CARE ORDER

The child is placed in the care of the local authority. It does not necessarily mean that the child is away from home but the parental responsibility is shared by the local authority and the parents. In any dispute over the arrangements for the child, the local authority would have the final say. The local authority has the power to remove the child from home without applying for any other order. The care order lasts until the child is 18 unless the court discharges the order earlier.

The police also have separate powers to protect children, lasting up to seventy-two hours. During this time the designated police officer may apply for an emergency protection order.

Going to court

If there is a decision to go to court, this should be planned as carefully as possible. The decision is taken by the local authority, usually after consultation with other agencies, and after taking advice from their law departments. The process will start in the local Family Proceedings Court (the magistrates' court). When applying to the courts, the application must clearly identify the grounds for concern, and the proposed medium- and long-term future plans for the child.

If, as a child-care practitioner, you are called to act as a witness by the local authority, you are entitled to legal advice concerning your evidence from the local authority lawyer. If there is a conflict between you and the local authority, you must ask your own employer to arrange for legal advice from another lawyer, experienced in child-care proceedings.

As a general rule all professionals have a responsibility to disclose information to other *relevant* agencies where there is any suspicion that a child is being abused. It is important not to share this information with any other person or agency as doing so may leave you open to legal action. Any record may be subpoenaed by the courts for either civil or criminal proceedings. There are rules governing disclosure of documentation and confidentiality in court proceedings, and you should always gain legal advice in these situations.

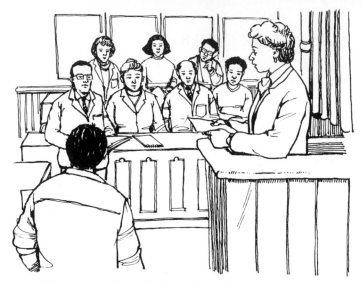

Child-care practitioners may be asked to give evidence in court

Local procedures

All child protection services are built around a document entitled *Working Together Under the Children Act (1989)*, published by the Department of Health in 1991. This important document issues general guidance about child protection procedures. The Area Child Protection Committee (ACPC) is then expected to define in more detail the procedures to be followed within each local area. These details will be published and issued to all professional agencies working in the area.

Activity

Discuss with your supervisor how you may find a copy of local procedures. Which agencies will be involved?

The ACPC carries executive responsibility for all child protection services in its area. It has to establish procedures, and will be expected to:

- monitor procedures
- identify significant issues arising from day-to-day casework
- arrange training
- promote liaison between the agencies
- review cases following death or serious injury.

The ACPC will publish an annual report, and will be regularly inspected by the Department of Health.

When there is concern about a child, all authorities will follow similar procedures, although there may be some differences in detail.

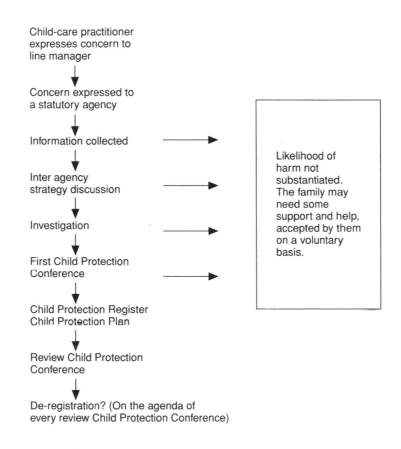

The child protection process

Referrals and investigations

An investigation of child abuse will often by triggered by a referral that may come from a number of different sources:

- the child may disclose information to an adult
- family or relatives, neighbours and other members of the public – some calls may be anonymous but still have to be investigated, although research suggests that the process will stop after the first inquiry

- professionals working with children from many different settings, health personnel based in the community and in hospital, teachers and child-care practitioners in schools, day-care centres and under-fives settings and voluntary agencies such as Childline.

To think about

You think a child might be being abused in the block of flats where you live. You have not witnessed any abuse, but are highly suspicious as the 3-year-old in the family always looks unhappy and neglected. What should you do? What range of feelings might you experience?

Once a referral has been made to social services, the police or the NSPCC, a consultation will take place to check if there is prior knowledge of the family, to decide whether there are grounds for an investigation, and what the roles of the agencies concerned in this investigation should be. It is never the role of the child-care practitioner to carry out an investigation.

The investigation will attempt to establish the truth in any allegation, to make a record of the allegations and the evidence, to assess the current risk to the child, to find out if there are continuing grounds for concern and whether protection procedures should be put in place, and possibly offer other services.

The investigation is the responsibility of the child protection investigative team, which may comprise a police officer and a social worker or a paediatrician and social worker. All have received special training and are skilled in child abuse cases. Their first task is to establish contact with the parents of the child, and any other key carers in the child's life. They will then interview the child in the child's home if this is not a threatening place. This may be repeated later at a specialist centre using video equipment, which may be used in evidence in criminal proceedings.

Immediate steps could be taken to protect the child if it was thought the child was at risk. This would nearly always be on a voluntary basis, while further investigation is undertaken, although emergency orders could be sought. There is often less urgency in cases of emotional and sexual abuse where a softly-softly approach might yield better results, and the damage has already been inflicted, than in cases of physical abuse where the risk of injury might be escalating. If it is thought that abuse is taking place within the family, all other siblings would be seen and interviewed. The investigation may require a medical examination to take place. This will usually be carried out in a hospital by a paediatrician. As this may be used in evidence it will have to be very thorough, and may involve an internal examination and the taking of various swabs and samples.

The alleged abuser will be interviewed, usually at a police station. This interview will be tape-recorded and may be used in evidence. It is very rare for young children to be interviewed without their parents' knowledge and consent. The investigation would require collecting as much information as possible about the child, the family and the alleged abuser from other professional workers, as all

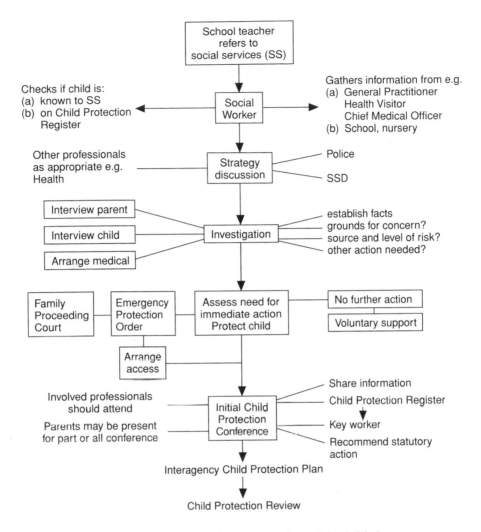

An outline procedure for investigating a case of possible child abuse

agencies have a general duty to assist the local authority. If the parents are uncooperative, a child assessment order may be sought from the Court. A Guardian *ad litem* (see page 101) might be appointed to protect the child's interests at this time. A child able to understand the concept of assessment and medical examination may withhold consent.

Following this investigation, if there is no cause for concern, the person with parental responsibility, the child and the referrer are informed in writing. If there are grounds for concern there will be a formal child protection conference.

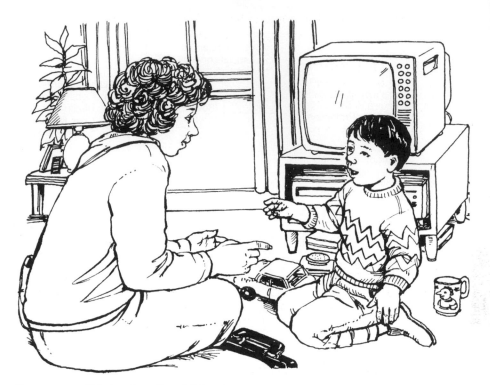

Key carers will interview the child at home

The child protection conference

The document *Working Together Under the Children Act, 1989*, issued by the Department of Health, recommends that the conference should be held within eight working days, with a maximum of fifteen days. Social services are responsible for calling the conference, which is not called to apportion blame but to:

■ exchange information
■ decide on the level of risk
■ decide if the child needs to be placed on the register
■ make some forward-thinking decisions for the benefit of the family and the protection of the child.

Conferences require a number of different agencies to be present before decisions can be made. Specialists such as child psychiatrists and experts in family law, who may not know the family previously, may be called to give advice.

As a child-care practitioner you may be required to attend a child protection conference to present an observation you have made of the child, or an assessment of any recent changes in the child's behaviour. You will not be asked for opinions but only for objective evidence, and this is where your observations and record keeping will be most valuable. You may be sent an agenda in advance and the

Department of Health has devised a checklist that you should receive prior to a conference but is not always received in time. This will give you basic information about:

- why the conference has been called
- who will be present
- the task to be accomplished
- the decisions to be made
- definitions of abuse
- criteria for registration
- information concerning local procedures.

At the very least, it is useful to know why the conference is being called and what is expected of you at the conference.

Parents and carers will be invited to attend the conference for at least part of the time and will be given the opportunity to express their views themselves or through a representative. The child may also attend the conference if he or she is thought to be old enough to understand the proceedings.

If the conference decides the child is suffering or is likely to suffer significant harm, the conference will register the child under one or several categories. It will appoint and name a key worker, and recommend a core group of professionals to be involved in a child protection plan. A review date will be set. Parents should be encouraged to participate in child protection conferences and professionals should inform parents of the information that they are going to present. No additional information should be given at the last minute.

Activity
Within the bounds of confidentiality, ask your supervisor or line manager if he or she has attended a child protection conference. Ask what procedures were used and whether the parents present. What briefing and de-briefing did they receive?

The child protection register

This is held by the social services Department and maintained on computer. Children can be placed on the register who are judged to be ' at risk' but only after the decision is taken by a fully quorate case conference where all professional participants have been allowed to express a view. The decision will reflect the perceived risk of future abuse as well as past abuse and it is possible to place an unborn baby on the register if someone in the family is a known abuser. The register provides a central record of children known to be 'at risk', so that agencies who are concerned about an individual family can check their current status. Access to the register is usually restricted to senior officers of any agency, but making this check is an essential part of professional responsibility. Anyone contacting the keeper of the register by telephone would be called back with the information asked for to ensure that security and confidentiality is maintained. The register should indicate under what categories of abuse or neglect the child has been registered, and the position should be regularly reviewed.

The register should contain the:

- full name of the child, and any aliases or 'known by' names
- address, sex, date of birth, ethnic and religious group
- full names of those who have care of the child, together with information about who has parental responsibility
- details of the GP
- school, nursery, playgroup etc. attended by the child
- date when the child was placed on the register
- categories of abuse under which the child is registered
- name and address of the key worker
- date for review
- legal status of the child (any orders which affect the parents' rights etc.)

Any changes to the information require the data to be amended and all other agencies to be informed. There should also be procedures to deal with situations where children go missing, any major incident affecting a child, or when any child moves to another authority. As part of the continuing action to protect the child, a core group will be appointed under the leadership of a key worker (generally the social worker). This group will draw up a detailed child protection plan, and may undertake more thorough assessment. The core group will:

- attempt to establish effective communication
- identify the roles of each agency
- set time limits and the timetable for reviews and meetings
- define contact arrangements with the family
- make alternative provisional plans.

Activity

You have attended a conference because a child in your establishment has been sexually abused by a family friend. As part of the child protection plan you have been asked to monitor the child's behaviour and emotional development, and keep detailed records.

1 How might you begin this task?
2 How would you ensure the co-operation of the parent/carer?
3 Identify possible difficulties, and the strategies you might use to overcome them.

Reviews and de-registration

Reviews should be held at least six-monthly to re-assess the child protection plan or to take the decision to de-register the child. At least three agencies should be present for such a decision to be taken. The child may be removed from the register because:

- the risk of abuse has receded within the family
- the child has been placed away from home, and is no longer in contact with the abuser

- the abusing adult has left the household
- the child has moved to another area
- the child has reached 18, married, or has died.

De-registration does not necessarily mean that social work support is not needed by the family.

The registration of child-care practitioners

There has been much debate and discussion over the last ten years about the lack of procedures governing the employment of nannies in private homes. Child-care practitioners working in day-care, nursery and school settings are required to submit to a rigorous application procedure, supplying references and undergoing police checks. Those working in private homes are not necessarily checked to the same degree of rigour.

There is a strong movement towards a child-care register, whose primary aim is to protect children. Any person wishing to work with children, whether trained or untrained, would have to be seen to be a suitable person before being placed on the register, following police and medical checks, and the provision of references. There would be a professional Code of Conduct, and any complaint upheld at a disciplinary hearing would result in removal from the register. This would be very similar to the register held for nursing and medical staff, but would differ in that it might not necessarily guarantee that the child-care practitioner had adequate experience or training.

Anyone can start a nanny agency and since 1995 agencies have not been required to obtain a licence to operate. The Department of Health recently stated that employing a nanny was a private contractual arrangement between the parents and the employee, and that it was up to the parent to make the checks on the person they employed. Parents often assume that the agency has made the checks, but this is not always the case.

The Federation of Recruitment and Employment services has a specialist child-care section of almost one hundred members (agencies) who all comply with a Code of Practice on placing nannies. This covers reference checking, interviewing and qualification checks. Any agency who breaches the code is subject to disciplinary procedures. If you wish to register with an agency, you would be advised to check that the agency belongs to this federation, and certainly advise any parent to use only federation agencies.

The Employment Agencies Act Regulations state that agencies must make sure that candidates are suitable for any job for which they are put forward. For nannies, this would include taking up references. In a television programme in July

1997, a reporter pretending to seek employment as a nanny, visited several agencies. Without exception, she was granted interviews with families before her references (which were false) were checked. Two families offered her a job. The Playpen Campaign has been initiated to push for legislation for a national register by a mother, Cheryl Winton – whose child was brain-damaged by an unqualified nanny after being shaken as a baby – and by Anne Waddington, a barrister who specialises in child protection. At least if there was a child-care register, prospective employers should be able to ascertain that the candidate for the job has no reason not to be registered. Some recent research by the Psychological Research Foundation in a survey covering 561 British mothers found that:

- only 49 per cent asked to see written evidence of any vocational and educational qualifications, including photocopies, and of that percentage only 8 per cent asked to see the original documents
- the mothers had hired 2,278 nannies, an average of just over 4 each
- one mother had hired and fired 31 nannies, and another had employed and sacked 15 nannies and of the remaining 24 per cent the mothers had hired 5 or more nannies each
- although 75 per cent required the nanny to drive a car, less than 1 in 3 asked to see the current driver's licence.

Unhappily, as there is a shortage of people wanting to work in private homes, this situation may well continue. Employers tend to turn a blind eye to minor misdemeanours as they are so reliant on nannies to enable them to continue their own professional careers.

KEY TERMS

You need to know what these words and phrases mean. Go back through the chapter and make sure that you understand:

anti-discrimination practices
Area Child Protection Committees
 (ACPCs)
care order, child assessment order
 and emergency protection order
child advocacy centres
the Children Act, 1989
de-registration
disclosure

parental responsibility
partnership with parents
recovery order and supervision order
registration of child-care
 practitioners
residence order
significant harm
statutory responsibility

Resources

Children's Legal Centre Briefing: *Children's Rights after Cleveland; The Children Act 1989;* and *The UN Convention on the Rights of the Child* (leaflets)
Cobley, C., *Child Abuse and the Law,* Cavendish Publishing Ltd, 1995

Department of Health, *An Introduction to the Children Act, 1989*, HMSO, 1991 (leaflet); *An Introductory Guide for the NHS: the Children Act, 1989,* 1992 (free leaflet); *Children and Young People on Child Protection Registers, Year ending 31.3.96*, Government Statistical Service, 1996 (frec leaflet)

Donnelly, C. (Ed), *What are Children's Rights?*, Independence, 1996

Jenkins, P., 'When child abuse is legal' in *Nursery World*: 9.3.95

Levy, A. (Ed), *Focus on Child Abuse, Medical, Legal and Social Work Perspectives*, Hawkesmere Ltd, 1989

Lyon, C. and de Cruz, P., *Child Abuse,* Jordan, 1993

Newell, P., *The UN Convention and Children's Rights in the UK*, National Children's Bureau, 1991

Stainton, Rogers W. and Roche, J., *Children's Welfare and Children's Rights: a Practical Guide to the Law*, Hodder and Stoughton, 1994

3 DEFINING ABUSE

During your career as a child-care practitioner you will probably come into contact with more than one child who is being abused. You will find this distressing and as a professional person, you will need to have some idea why this happens, how to recognise abuse, what procedures to follow, and how to help the child and the family. Child abuse may be difficult to define but a clear understanding is necessary so that you may act with confidence when working with vulnerable children.

The needs of children

During your training you will have looked at the needs of children, so as to ensure optimum growth and development. If these needs are not met, children will not thrive. These needs are shown in the diagram on page 43 – based on studies by Maslow (Oliver, 1993).

Defining child abuse

There are some commonly accepted definitions of child abuse, but when looking at a number of local authority child protection documents you will see a variety of definitions. The broad categories are neglect, physical abuse and injury, emotional abuse and sexual abuse, but all these categories overlap and interconnect.

One way of defining abuse is Kidscape's statement: 'Child abuse is
- making a child feel unwanted, ugly, worthless, guilty, unloved
- being physically violent to a child
- exploiting a child sexually
- failing to provide the things needed for a child to grow.'

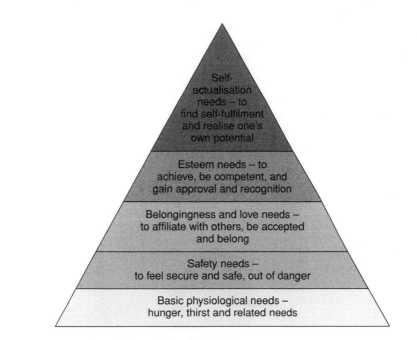

Maslow's hierarchy of the needs of children

Activity

Obtain a copy of your local authority's child protection procedures. How are the areas of abuse defined?

A report, *Childhood Matters*, published by the National Commission of Inquiry into the Prevention of Child Abuse defines abuse as: 'Child abuse consists of anything which individuals, institutions or processes do or fail to do, which directly or indirectly harms children or damages their prospects of safe and healthy development into childhood'.

To think about

Should everybody be obliged by law to report suspected child abuse? Do you think a national campaign showing violent distressing images of abused children raises public awareness and encourages people to report suspected abuse?

PHYSICAL ABUSE AND INJURY

Physical abuse of children is intentional, non-accidental use of physical force and violence, resulting in hurting, injuring or destroying the child. It includes poisoning. Most at risk are under 2-year-olds but children of all ages suffer from it.

NEGLECT

This failure by the parents/carers to provide adequately for the needs and safety of their children is not always intentional. Some parents/carers put their own needs and interests first and neglect the child, while others might be unwell or unable to cope. All children are vulnerable, but the pre-school child is most at risk. Neglect, thought to be five times more prevalent than physical abuse (Wolock and Horowitz, 1984; Young 1981), is difficult to diagnose, as it has to continue for quite a long time before the effects are visible. It is not only the very dirty, hungry child who is neglected – the term includes abandoning children for periods of time, emotional and educational neglect, and not providing a secure environment. There have been several reported incidents of parents going on holiday and leaving their children inadequately cared for.

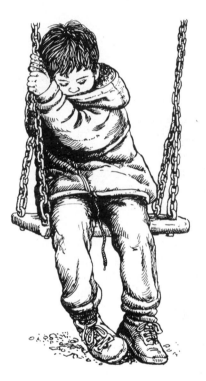

Neglect may be five times more prevalent than physical abuse

SEXUAL ABUSE

This is the 'involvement of dependent, developmentally immature children or adolescents in sexual activities that they do not truly comprehend, to which they are unable to give informed consent, or that violate the social taboos of family roles. In other words it is the use of children by adults for sexual gratification' (Schechter and Roberge, 1976). It can occur in any age group with boys or girls.

EMOTIONAL ABUSE

Children of any age group may be exposed to constant criticism and hostility, and lack of affection and warmth. They may be rejected or extremely over-protected. They often suffer from poor self-esteem and lack confidence.

As well as these four broad categories of abuse defined by the Department of Health there are other terms you need to be familiar with.

FAILURE TO THRIVE

Failure to thrive occurs when a child fails to gain weight or to grow and achieve his or her expected weight and height. Children who have no medical or physical reason not to develop normally, may fail to thrive resulting from a negative relationship with the parent/carer. This is likely to be picked up in the younger age group, when children are regularly monitored and attending health clinics.

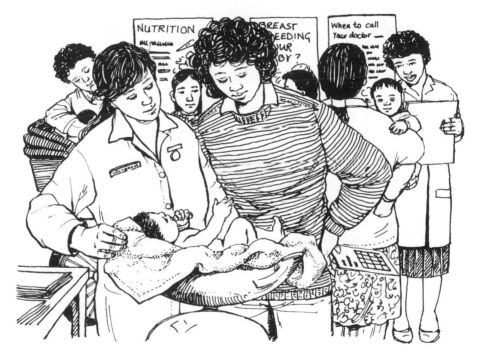

Regular monitoring may reveal failure to thrive

Activity

Obtain and discuss documentation used by health care professionals to monitor children's growth and development.

ORGANISED ABUSE

This generally refers to sexual abuse and may involve physical injury. There will be a number of perpetrators and a number of abused children. There is an element of deliberate planning. It may refer to a paedophile ring, prostitution or the involvement of children in the production of pornographic material, and may include an element of ritual or the occult. This might be used to instil fear in the victims and so ensure secrecy. The extent of 'ritual' or 'Satanic' abuse is disputed.

To think about
How appropriate is it to 'celebrate' Halloween with very young children?

MUNCHAUSEN SYNDROME BY PROXY

This syndrome is used to describe a physchological condition where a parent fabricates a child's illness, seeking many different medical opinions and inducing symptoms in the child to deceive the doctors. Munchausen syndrome describes adults who present themselves with symptoms of an illness so as to receive attention for themselves, Munchausen by proxy extends this to the child. The parent wishes to be looked upon as a good parent, caring and attentive to his or her child.

GRAVE CONCERN

This was a term used by the Department of Health in 1991 who stated that the term 'should not be used lightly and should be needed only in exceptional circumstances for children whose situations do not currently fit the main four categories. This may be where there is an explicit and serious concern that the child is not developing as would be expected (and all medical causes have been eliminated) or there is a sudden unexplained change in the child's normal behaviour pattern. If the cause of the child's condition is later established as fitting one of the above categories, a case conference should amend the cause of registration'.

SIGNIFICANT HARM

This concept is embodied within the Children Act, 1989, Section 31 (2): 'A court may only make a care order or supervision order if it is satisfied:
(a) that the child concerned is suffering or is likely to suffer, significant harm
(b) that the harm or likelihood of harm, is attributable to:
(i) the care given to the child, or likely to be given to him if the order were not made, not being what it would be reasonable to expect a parent to give him
(ii) the child's being beyond parental control'.
The guide on page 47 considers the amount of harm by looking at the effect the abuse has had on the individual child's normal development.

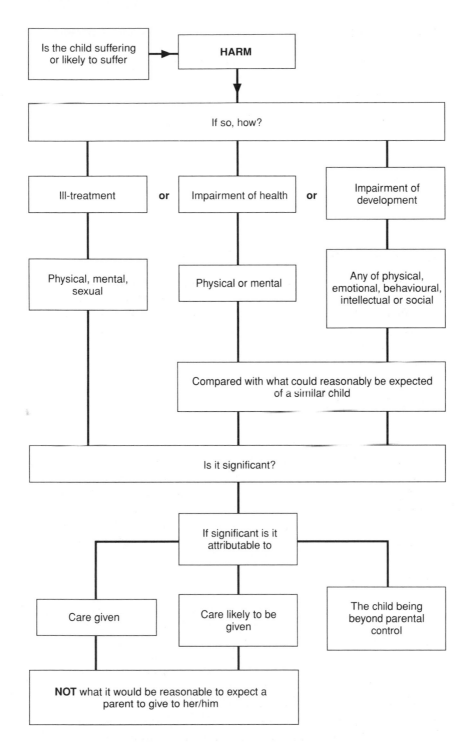

Significant harm criteria

As a generalisation, the more abusive the child's experience, the greater deviation from normal growth and development can be expected. Abusing a child can include many categories: a child who is physically neglected may well be starved of love as well as food; a child who is sexually abused may also be physically injured and emotionally upset. This overlap will become apparent when we look at the recognition of abuse in chapter 4.

To think about
Would you extend any of the definitions of abuse and neglect?

Family abductions

The removal of a child by one parent without the consent of the other is an extremely distressing experience for the child and the parent who loses the child.

The number of children involved in these cases appears to be growing due to:
- cheaper and more accessible global travel
- free movement of people within the European community and the reduction of border controls
- increased numbers of mixed marriages/relationships, without a clear understanding of the cultural and religious customs of the other partner
- courts now making court orders defining residence only if it is better for the child than making no order.

Parents who are married share parental responsibility for their child, including the decision as to where the child should live. The law does not require them to consult with one another in exercising their parental responsibility. Each may act alone. It is within the law for a married parent to remove a child from the home without the consent of the other parent, providing they do not remove the child to outside the UK.

Where there is disagreement between parents, an application can be made to the court for a residence order stating where the child should live, or possibly an injunction preventing one parent removing the child from the care of the other. The same circumstances apply to divorced couples where no court order has been made. When a couple is in a partnership rather than a marriage, the father will have parental responsibility only if there is a parental responsibility agreement with the mother, a parental responsibility under Section 4 of the Children Act, or a residence order. Unless any of the above circumstances exist, it is unlawful for an unmarried father to remove the child from the mother.

If you are working in an establishment, you need to be extremely careful to hand over the children in your care only to named and known carers, with the authority of the parent (see the nursery start form, page 50). Never allow a child to go with someone about whom you are doubtful, however plausible they may appear.

UNIVERSITY OF LONDON UNION
DAY NURSERY START FORM

1 Medical details

i) Please give detils of your child's vaccination programme:

_____

_____

ii) Please give details of any infectious diseases and child ailments:

_____

_____

iii) Please give details of allergies, any allergic condition, or food intolerance:

_____

_____

iv) Please give details of any serious illness that your child may have had, to include any hospital admissions:

_____

_____

v) Any further or other information which may be significant to your child's health and welfare:

_____

_____

2 Doctor's name: _____

Address: _____

_____

Telephone: _____

3 Health visitor's name: _____

Address: _____

_____

Telephone: _____

4 Social worker's name: _____

Address: _____

_____

Telephone: _____

5 Consent for administration of drugs.

I/we give my/our consent for the administratin of basic first aid treatment (no prescribed medicines) to be given to my/our child/children by the nursery staff; and also for my/our child/children to be treated in hospital in an emergency, at the doctor's discretion.

An example of a day nursery start form

I/we will not allow my/our child/children to be administered the following drug(s) or treatment(s) under any circumstances:

_____

_____

Full name of child (CAPITALS): _____

_____

Signed: _____ (Parent or legal guardian)
Date: _____

6 I/we hereby give permission for my/our child to be taken off the premises under the supervision of a responsible member of nursery staff:

Full name of child (CAPITALS): _____

_____

Signed: _____ (Parent or legal guardian)

7 Please provide names and addresses of 2 people other than yourself or your partner, who we can contact in an emergency if we are unable to contact either parent/guardian.

i) Name: _____
Relationship to child if any: _____
Daytime contact number: _____

ii) Name: _____
Relationship to child if any: _____
Daytime contact number: _____

8 Name(s) of any person(s) allowed to collect your child:

_____

_____

_____

NB: Anyone not named here will be refused acces to your child unless we have received confirmation from you or your partner in person.

9 Name(s) of any person(s) NOT allowed to collect your child:

_____

_____

_____

10 Declaration:

I/we have read the regulations governing the admission of children to the University of London Union Day Nursery and I/we agree to conform to and comply with these regulations.
Signature(s) of parent/guardian: _____

_____

Date: _____

If you are working in a private home, and one parent fears the child may be abducted by the other one you should advise the parent to:

- encourage the separated parent to remain part of the child's life, keeping in touch by letter and telephone, giving the parent regular information about the child's progress and development
- seek counselling and support services
- seek a court order containing a restriction against removal
- always make sure the child is accompanied when away from home
- keep all important information concerning the child in a safe, accessible place as quick action might be needed in an emergency – this information might include photographs of children and parents, copies of court orders, full details of the child's passport, telephone numbers of the police and solicitor, and full details of the potential abductor
- consult a solicitor with specific expertise
- keep the child's passport in a safe place, either in a bank or with a solicitor
- prevent the other parent obtaining a birth certificate: this can be done by contacting St Catherine's House in London
- arrange for contact visits to be supervised, and do not allow the child to leave the country on a contact visit.

The Hague and the European Conventions, ratified in August 1986, secured the return of the child to the child's country of habitual residence, so that disputes can be resolved by the courts. There is no requirement under the Conventions that the welfare of the child is paramount, and the merits of the case are not examined. Where a child is abducted to a country which is not subject to the Conventions, proceedings will have to be started in that country. This is a complex area, and if you should be involved in any aspect you should seek further advice.

To think about

Do you think marriage between two people from different countries, with conflicting belief systems, is usually successful?

Exploitation of children

CHILD PROSTITUTION

Prostitution is defined as the provision of sexual services in exchange for some form of payment, which may range from money, drink or drugs to goods or provision of a basic need, such as shelter or food. Child prostitution includes both boys and girls under the age of 16 years. Home Office figures show that between 1989 and 1993 nearly 1,500 children under 18 were convicted for offences relating to prostitution, and a further 1,800 were cautioned. Cautions of girls between 10 years and 16 years rose by nearly 50 per cent and convictions by 10 per cent over this period of time. Factors leading to this increase are:

- poverty and gaps in the benefit system leading to homelessness and family conflict
- increasing family break ups and reconstituted family structures which sometimes lead to emotionally damaged children, often starved of affection at home, and subsequently taken into care
- abused children
- inadequate sex education policies
- inadequate social policies to ensure that children in care are properly supervised and protected
- drug and alcohol abuse
- the law relating to pimps and clients of under-age prostitutes appears to discriminate against the children, rather than the adults
- the notion of life in a big city may appeal to young immature people who then become trapped by adults preying on them.

CHILD EMPLOYMENT

The main areas of employment for children in this country are:

- family businesses
- newspaper rounds

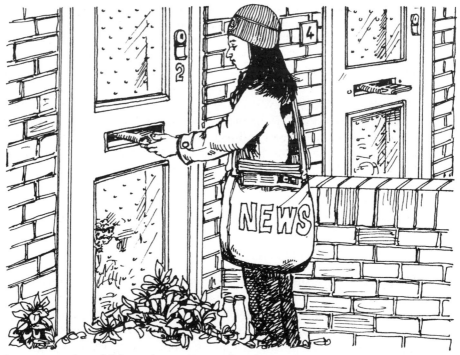

Laws governing child employment are often ignored

- shop work
- cleaning
- baby sitting
- running errands.

All these teach children responsibility and independence, but the danger is that the children are exploited by being paid very little, and are expected to work too many hours which erodes their ability to concentrate and make progress at school and to enjoy their childhood. In some areas of employment they may be at risk from lack of training or awareness of health and safety issues. Studies appear to indicate that children and families are not aware of the laws concerning child employment. The laws regarding employment of young people may be more rigorous if Britain signs the European Social Charter.

Female genital mutilation

Women who have undergone genital mutilation are often more likely to wish their own daughters to suffer this procedure, seeing it as culturally correct and in their daughters' best interests. Child-care practitioners should be alert to the possibility of mutilation when working with members from a community known to practice genital mutilation extensively, and the risk is higher if elderly female relatives are part of the family group.

Mutilation may occur from the first week of birth up to the age of 12, using a variety of implements, frequently unsterilised, without anaesthesia. The practice is widespread in many parts of Africa, Asia and the Middle East.

The practice has been illegal in the UK since 1985. It may result in serious health risks to the child, including shock, urine retention, tetanus, loss of blood and pelvic infection as well as infertility and complications during pregnancy and childbirth. Western countries have been looked upon as racist in their disapproval of this practice by the countries where it is carried out. In the UK anyone involved in multi-disciplinary child protection work has a duty to work in partnership with the parents as long as it is consistent with the child's welfare and to address issues concerning race and gender which might affect the way a child might best be helped. It is clear, however, that legal steps must be taken to prevent a child being mutilated and social workers may seek an emergency protection order or a 'prohibited steps' order to prevent the child being sent out of the country. If it is impossible to dissuade the parents from mutilating the child, child protection procedures might be invoked.

Paedophiles

People who sexually abuse children are called paedophiles. Usually male but sometimes female, they come from all classes, professions, races and religions. They are not immediately identifiable as they keep their sexual life secret. In May 1997, a paedophile ring was discovered composed of members of the St John's Ambulance Brigade, usually regarded as people one can trust implicitly. Paedophiles can be any member of the general population and are only identified after disclosure or discovery. They prey mainly on children they know and often go to great lengths to get on good terms with a particular family, to infiltrate games clubs for children, or to make themselves indispensable to schools. Single parent families are particularly vulnerable as the mothers can become isolated and lonely, and the children may not have a male role model living at home.

In the United States, in New Jersey, after the sexual assault, kidnapping and killing of a child named Megan a law was passed requiring courts to inform local people when a convicted sex offender is released or paroled into their community. This campaign became a national crusade, and 41 states have followed New Jersey, invoking 'Megan's Law'.

To think about
Do you think Megan's Law contravenes civil liberties?

In Wales in November 1996 and in London in 1997, parents of children attending local primary schools were issued with warnings about convicted paedophiles who had moved into the area that contained descriptions of their appearance.

The government has now introduced a national register of convicted child sex offenders to enable the police to track and supervise such people and to check on potential child-care employees with unsupervised access to young children. Unfortunately this does not include paedophiles who have not been convicted. Less than half the known paedophiles have registered their names and addresses with the police, even though discovery will lead to a heavy fine and/or imprisonment.

In July 1997, Camden ACPC in London issued guidelines entitled *Keeping Children and Young People Safe from Abuse* advising organisations to question job applicants about previous convictions, follow up references and contact child protection agencies if they believed someone may pose a threat. This is particularly relevant to small independent groups, who are not legally required to register with the local authority, such as small football clubs.

The NSPCC suggests that children are rarely picked at random and that paedophiles are skilled at identifying vulnerable children. They may target a child who is:

- too trusting
- seeking love or affection
- lonely or bereaved
- lacking in confidence
- bullied
- disabled or unable to communicate well
- in care, or away from home

- already a victim of abuse
- eager to succeed in activities, such as sport or other interests which may allow the child to be manipulated by a potential abuser.

Paedophiles often take time to groom children, leading them through a progression of activities from 'innocent' cuddling to an introduction to pornography, and finally to sexual activity using different ways of ensuring that the child remains silent.

Your suspicions might be aroused if someone from outside the family is taking too close an interest in a child in your care and the child appears to be uneasy in their presence, or even shows signs or behavioural indicators of abuse.

Bullying

Since the 1990s there has been increasing concern about bullying and the effect it has on children and their development. It has not always been seen as abuse, unless the effect on the child or the bullying is extreme. The Department for Education and Employment has issued a collection of circulars on matters concerning child protection, including bullying and in 1994 made a 'bullying pack' available to all schools. Dan Olweus, an expert in the prevention of bullying, defines bullying as involving:

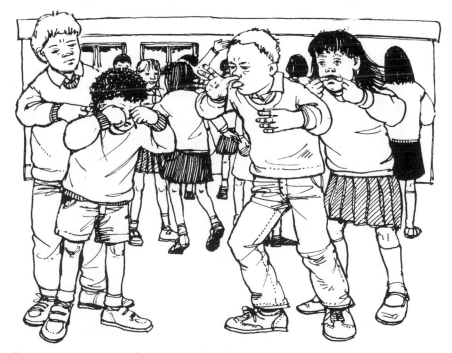

Bullying can cause long-lasting emotional scars

- deliberate hostility and aggression towards the victim
- a victim who is weaker and less powerful than the bully or bullies
- an outcome which is always painful and distressing to the victim.

It can be physical, verbal, emotional, racist and/or sexual. In its extreme form, it can lead to suicide in young people, and is the main cause for school refusal. It can result in emotional scars which remain for life.

Few school children escape coming into contact with a bully during their school days. Children who bully and seek power over others have problems similar to those of abusive parents and need help and understanding. The child who is bullied may show few physical signs, although there may be scratches, cuts and bruises which he or she is reluctant to explain.

The bully will often pick on a particular child who may be different in some way, either physically such as having poor co-ordination or speech or language difficulties or culturally such as belonging to a different ethnic or religious group from the majority of pupils.

Bullying is rare among under-5s, but can occur, even though they are usually well supervised at all times. In the infant school, some forms of bullying may take place, such as name calling, fighting, excluding a child from his or her peer group, sending to Coventry, and racial abuse.

Activity
How would you, as a child-care practitioner, manage a situation in a playground where a 7 year-old is taunting a younger child with obscene racist comments?

There are some behavioural indicators in children under 8 years of age. Children who are bullied may be:
- reluctant or refusing to attend school or nursery
- saying they feel unwell in the mornings
- coming home with torn clothes
- hungry, having had their lunch stolen
- withdrawn, unhappy or showing signs of poor self-esteem
- crying frequently, and waking with nightmares
- aggressive, or starting to bully other children
- reluctant to talk about what is happening to them.

To think about
Why do some children bully others? How can you help the bully in the infant school to recognise and stop this hurtful behaviour?

Activity
Looking back to your schooldays, were there any times when you were bullied? How did it make you feel? Did you ever become a bully yourself? Why do you think that was?

A recent article in a newspaper suggested that many 'Captains of industry' had been bullies at school, treading ruthlessly on the feelings and hopes of other people in their pursuit of power and achievement.

Children who abuse children

During the 1990s there has been increasing concern about children who are violent towards each other, sometimes causing death, as in the case of James Bulgar, a 2 year-old who was enticed away from a shopping centre by two boys of 9 and 10, and then tied up and stoned to death on a railway line, and a young girl who was killed by three other female teenagers at a fair. Children have also attacked and killed adults, as in the stabbing of Philip Lawrence and the gang rape and attempted killing of an Austrian tourist. Horrific as these isolated events are, of equal concern to child-care practitioners is the sexual abuse of children by other children.

A committee of enquiry set up by NCH Action for Children, reporting in 1992, found that up to 1 in 3 abusers were under the age of 18. A treatment centre at the Tavistock Clinic in London is currently working with 76 children. Children as young as 8 years old have been assessed and the clinic receives enquiries relating to children as young as 4. Ninety-one per cent of the abusers have been abused themselves, three quarters of them sexually. It was proposed that many of the children may have been exposed to pornographic material.

It is very difficult for the general public and many professional people to comprehend and believe that children can be sexually abusive towards one another, but failure to admit that this occurs will result in many more children suffering abuse.

To think about
What do you think is the main motivation behind children sexually abusing other children? What would you see as normal sexual experimentation?

Statistics

According to the NSPCC, an estimated 150 to 200 children die each year in England and Wales following incidents of abuse or neglect. Thousands more suffer long-term emotional and psychological problems because of ill treatment by their parents or those looking after them. More than 20,000 children a year tell Childline that they have been physically or sexually abused. Childline's report (1993/1994) states that they received:

- 10,942 calls concerning sexual abuse
- 10,028 calls concerning physical abuse

- 495 calls concerning emotional abuse
- 181 calls about neglect
- 634 calls concerning fears of abuse.

Childline counselled 9,048 girls and 1,899 boys about sexual abuse. In 94 per cent of cases it was by a person the child knew – 56 per cent were in the immediate family. The father was the abuser in 32 per cent of cases with girls and 30 per cent with boys. Counsellors identified 16 calls, mainly from girls, which talked about organised abuse, including prostitution.

The *Independent* reported in September 1995, that more than 5,000 under-age girls were working as prostitutes in Britain, and the number caught soliciting had doubled since 1990.

Figures published by the Department of Health, for the year ending 31 March, 1996, reveal that there were approximately 32,000 children on the Child Protection Register in England, a decrease of 7 per cent compared with the previous year.

Approximately 28,000 names were added to the register during the year showing a similar decrease of 7 per cent. During the year 30,000 children were de-registered. In the year 1994–95, registrations and de-registrations were both about 30,000.

In the year 1995–96 there were 44,100 children who were the subject of initial child protection conferences, 64 per cent of whom were placed on the register. In 82 per cent of registrations, it was the first time ever that the child's name was placed on a register. A similar number of girls and boys were added to the register overall, and slightly more boys than girls were de-registered.

- 40 per cent of registrations were children considered at risk of physical injury, 54 per cent of whom were boys.
- 33 per cent of registrations related to risk of neglect.
- 22 per cent of registrations related to the risk of sexual abuse, 61 per cent of whom were girls.

For a report issued by The Gulbenkian Foundation in 1995 on the incidence of violence to children see page 59. The report, *Childhood Matters,* was a two-year evidence-gathering exercise, involving over ten thousand individuals and organisations. They received over a thousand letters from survivors of child abuse. Of these 80 per cent said they had been sexually abused. Only 32 per cent said they had told anyone, and 13 per cent had never revealed what had happened. The evidence showed the abuse often began at pre-school age and continued well into adolescence. It estimated the annual cost of abuse at one billion pounds, at a conservative estimate, but was impossible to assess accurately because of the long-term effects of abuse.

A Hackney study, *Links Between Domestic Violence and Child Abuse,* showed that half the women killed each year were killed by partners, and 100,000 women each year seek medical help for injuries caused by partners. A violent crime survey, conducted by the Home Office in 1989, showed that 25 per cent of all assaults recorded by the police are domestic violence offences and around 10 to 15 per cent of cases were of violence against the person.

In an NCH Action for Children study in 1994 a quarter of the mothers said that their violent partners had also physically assaulted their children. Several said that

The extent of violence involving children

Children are far more often victims of violence than perpetrators of violence, and certain groups of children, including disabled children and some ethnic groups, are particularly at risk. One of the most disturbing social statistics is that the risk of homicide for babies under the age of one is almost four times as great as for any other age group. There is increasing knowledge of and sensitivity to violence to children – in particular to sexual abuse and to bullying and other violence in institutions; it is not possible to tell whether the incidence of these forms of violence has increased or become more visible. There are problems about building any accurate picture of violence to children within families, but the most recent UK research shows that a substantial minority of children suffer severe physical punishment; most children are hit by their parents, up to a third of younger children more than once a week.

Only a very small proportion of children

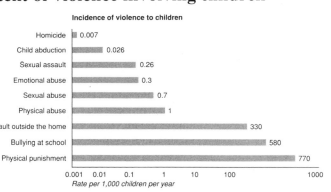

Incidence of violence to children

	Rate per 1,000 children per year
Homicide	0.007
Child abduction	0.026
Sexual assault	0.26
Emotional abuse	0.3
Sexual abuse	0.7
Physical abuse	1
Assault outside the home	330
Bullying at school	580
Physical punishment	770

– mostly male but with an increasing minority of young women – get involved in committing violent offences. Very roughly, four per 1,000 young people aged between 10 and 18 are cautioned or convicted for offences involving violence against the person.

In terms of trends it appears that children's involvement in some but not all crimes of violence in the UK has increased over the last decade. But in comparison with the USA, overall levels of interpersonal violence in the UK are very low, and there is recent evidence that in comparison with some European countries, levels of self-reported violence by children in the UK are also low.

A Gulbenkian Foundation report

the children had been sexually abused. More than five in six of the mothers thought that the children had been affected by the violence in the longer term. Many of the children showed signs and behaviour indicators of emotional abuse.

A recent leaflet from NCH Action for Children states that in March 1994 there were 9,600 children registered under the sexual abuse category on child protection registers – just over a quarter of all cases registered.

Activity

Continue to read your newspaper and professional magazines, noting and recording any statistical information. Looking at the separate areas of abuse, identify any upward or downward trends. If you have access to the Internet, compare the figures in the USA with those of the UK.

The problems of definition

Child Protection: Messages from Research, published by HMSO, 1995, has made the following points.

- 'Child abuse is difficult to define, but clear parameters for intervention are necessary if professionals are to act with confidence to protect vulnerable children.
- 'Thresholds which legitimise action on the part of child protection agencies appear as the most important components of any definition of child abuse.
- 'The research evidence suggests that authoritative knowledge about what is known to be bad for children should play a greater part in drawing these thresholds.
- 'A large number of children in need live in contexts in which their health and development are neglected. For these children it is the corrosiveness of long-term emotional, physical and occasionally sexual maltreatment that causes psychological impairment or even significant harm.
- 'Instances of child sexual abuse may not conform to general findings about child protection. For example, minor single incidents can damage children and thresholds and criminal statutes tend to be clearer than is found when dealing with physical abuse.'

Defining child abuse is not an exact concept. Thresholds, in particular, can be subjective. A threshold is the point when a child generates sufficient concern to be deemed in need of protection, and the child protection agencies become involved. For example, when does smacking become hitting? When does demonstrative affection become a sexual assault? You will need to bear all these points in mind if you are ever in the position of suspecting abuse of one of the children in your care.

KEY TERMS

You need to know what these words and phrases mean. Go back through the chapter and make sure that you understand:

abuse by children	female genital mutilation
child abuse	Munchausen syndrome by proxy
child employment	neglect
child prostitution	organised abuse
domestic violence	paedophiles
emotional abuse	physical abuse and injury
failure to thrive	pornography
family abductions	

Resources

Benedict, H., *Stand Up for Yourself*, Hodder Headline, 1996
Bond, H., 'Mothers who abduct children' in *Nursery World*: 9.11.95

Bryant, Mole K., *Bullying*, Wayland, 1994

Childline, *Children and Racism: a Childline Study*, 1996

Children's Legal Centre Briefing, *Child Abduction* (information sheet)

Corke, S., 'A damaging cult', in *Nursery World*: 10.9.92

HMSO, *Child Protection: Messages from Research*, 1995

Kidscape, *Protect Children from Paedophiles*; *Stop Bullying*, 1996;

NCH Action for Children, *The Report of the Committee of Inquiry into Children and Young People who Sexually Abuse Other Children*, 1992

NSPCC, *Protecting Children from Sexual Abuse in the Community*, 1997

Reunite: a pack informing parents how to prevent abduction by an estranged parent is available from Reunite, PO Box 4, London WC1X 3DX. Telephone: 0171 404 8357. (£1.50, including postage and packing)

Walker, A., *Possessing the Secret of Joy*, Jonathan Cape, 1992

Wallace, W., 'Children who abuse children' in *Nursery World*: 6.7.95

4 RECOGNISING ABUSE

This chapter covers:
- Physical abuse and injury
- Neglect
- Emotional abuse
- Sexual abuse
- Failure to thrive
- Organised abuse
- Munchausen syndrome by proxy
- Female sexual abusers
- Resources

In general, when a child has been abused, more than one type of abuse or neglect is present. If a child has been a victim of physical or sexual abuse, it is important to consider the emotional effect on the child's intellectual development and behaviour: the whole child needs to be considered. In this chapter we will outline the various signs of abuse and neglect separately, but you must always be conscious of possible overlap. It is also important for you to remember that, although the injury may not be accidental, it may not have been the intention of the parent/carer to harm the child, but may have resulted from different cultural approaches to discipline.

To think about
In the past, physical punishment was used to control children, and this still occurs in many families. In what particular cultural groups and religions today might this be more prevalent?

In this chapter, we shall discuss many signs and indicators of abuse and neglect. You should always be cautious in your approach as sometimes there is an innocent explanation.

Physical abuse and injury

Physical abuse implies physically harmful action directed against a child; it is usually defined by any inflicted injury such as bruises, burns, head injuries, fractures, abdominal injuries or poisoning.

C.H. Kempe

Most children will suffer accidental injuries. Deciding what is accidental and what has been inflicted upon a child can be a very difficult process, testing the skills of experienced paediatricians. Many signs which might lead you to think that abuse had taken place, might be explained. For example, bald patches may occur if children frequently twist and pull their hair as a comfort habit. Fractures may occur in some children with specific medical conditions. It is, however, your responsibility to be alert to any unexplained or suspicious injury, making sure you record your concerns, reporting and discussing it with your line manager as soon as possible.

CASE STUDY

Chantal, an 18-month-old child of an Afro-Caribbean father and an English mother, was routinely admitted to a workplace nursery. The newly qualified key worker identified what she thought were bruises on Chantal's buttocks and reported this to her experienced line manager, who examined the child and reassured the child-care practitioner that the marks were Mongolian blue spot – an area of natural hyperpigmentation that occurs in many African, Afro-Caribbean and Asian babies at birth.

Having read this chapter, can you identify any other signs or indicators that might be open to the wrong interpretation?

PHYSICAL SIGNS

Injuries on the face, neck or head

- All bruises on the head or face of a small baby should be investigated. Toddlers may fall and bruise themselves on the forehead, cheekbone or chin, but bruises on the cheek are suspicious, particularly if they appear on each side. Bruises may be caused by slapping, showing a distinctive outline. Punching a child results in an injury less defined, except if the child is punched in the ear or the eye, where distinctive bruising will be seen. Bruises on the scalp may be difficult to see but are tender to touch. Bruising of the lips and gums may be caused by hitting or ramming a feeding bottle into the mouth of a crying baby.
- Bald patches may be seen on some children.
- Cigarette burns, which may appear anywhere on the face or body, are small circular burns frequently seen at different stages, suggesting frequent and repeated incidents.
- Small haemorrhages of the ear lobe are rarely accidental. Two black eyes would be suspicious, especially if there is no other injury to the head or face. Haemorrhages in the eye can sometimes be seen, but are often invisible unless an ophthalmoscope is used. These can last for up to four weeks after the injury.
- A direct blow to the head may fracture the skull. Shaking the child may lead to bleeding in the head, sometimes resulting in a coma or convulsions. Severe injuries to the head may produce damage to nerves, leading to a squint.
- A torn frenulum (the tongue attachment) is suspicious, but may occur when a child contracts whooping cough, although this is extremely rare.

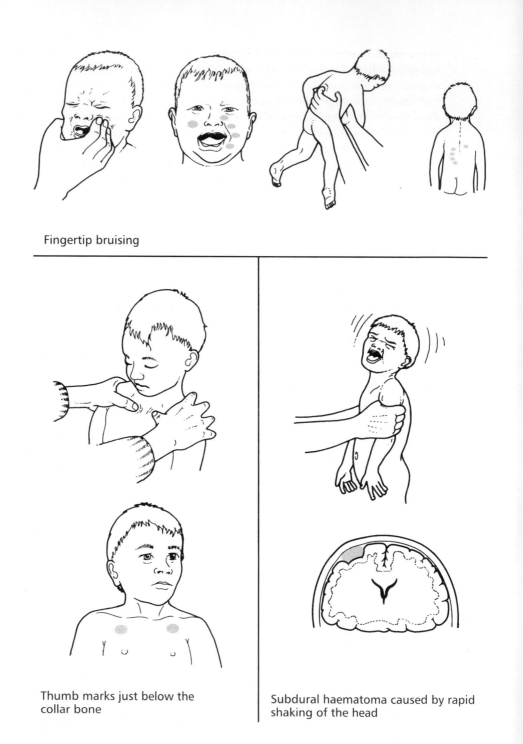

Fingertip bruising

Thumb marks just below the collar bone

Subdural haematoma caused by rapid shaking of the head

Examples of fingertip bruising, thumb marks and shaking

- Signs of injury on a neck should always be taken very seriously. This is a very rare site for accidental injury.

Injuries to the limbs and torso
- Fingertip bruising may be seen as a cluster of small bruises, like finger pressure marks often with the mark of the opposing thumb some distance away. This is seen where the child has been forcibly gripped, especially around the elbows and knees, on the trunk, and occasionally around the mouth. Thumb marks under the collar bones would indicate the child has been grasped and if on both sides, possibly shaken. Bruises on genitalia should always be regarded with great suspicion. Bruising anywhere on the body along a straight line would indicate being beaten with a belt, strap or stick. Bite marks will be seen as two semi-circular bruises. Care must be taken to distinguish between adult and child size bites. Kicking a child results in diffuse bruising, occasionally a mark of the footwear may be seen. Bruises seen when the skin is close to a bone are usually accidental, but those on soft tissue such as the cheeks, mouth and buttocks are more suspicious. Bruises are seen in 90 per cent of physically abused children. They go through a process of change from red/blue, often swollen, to purple, to green-brown/yellow as they age.
- Small children, particularly babies, who are unable to move a limb, should have this injury investigated. Fractures may be caused by a direct blow to the limb, or by grabbing and twisting the child's limb with some force.
- Scratches on the child's body may show fingernail marks.
- Injuries caused by scalds may be caused by 'dunking' the child in very hot water, leaving a high water mark. Hot liquids thrown at a child may produce scattered 'splash' burns. Hot liquid poured onto a child produces a broad linear mark. Marks on the soles of the feet might suggest 'dunking' a child on or near a fire. Burns on the buttocks are rarely accidental. Burns may also be caused by an iron or a hotplate, and these would show the telltale marks.

Some injuries are caused internally. Kicking or punching, resulting in injury to some organs of the body, such as liver, spleen or kidneys, can only be diagnosed by a doctor. Doctors investigating allegations of physical abuse will often call for a full skeletal X-ray. Children may also be physically abused by poisoning. This may be by medication, drugs, alcohol or other dangerous substances.

Activity
Tracey, aged 4 years, has been happily settled in your nursery class for the past two terms. Her parents divorced one year ago but Tracey and her mother receive a great deal of support from her large extended family. One morning Tracey arrives with both eyes bruised, a bruise on her neck and a red mark on her ear. She tells you that she fell off her bike.
  How do you react to this situation?

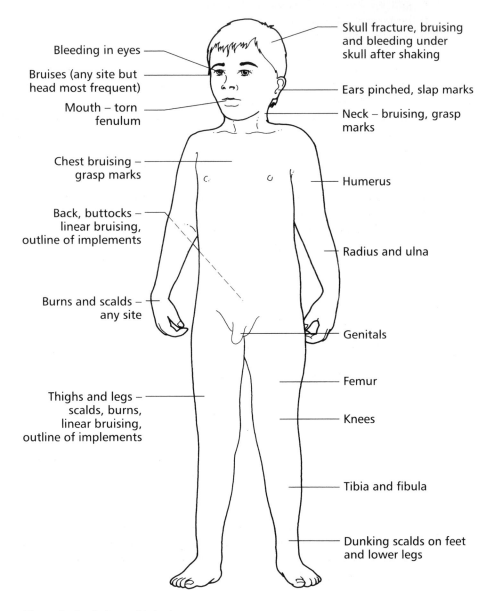

Bleeding in eyes

Bruises (any site but head most frequent)

Mouth – torn fenulum

Chest bruising – grasp marks

Back, buttocks – linear bruising, outline of implements

Burns and scalds – any site

Thighs and legs – scalds, burns, linear bruising, outline of implements

Skull fracture, bruising and bleeding under skull after shaking

Ears pinched, slap marks

Neck – bruising, grasp marks

Humerus

Radius and ulna

Genitals

Femur

Knees

Tibia and fibula

Dunking scalds on feet and lower legs

The principal sites of injuries

BEHAVIOURAL INDICATORS OF PHYSICAL ABUSE

Physical abuse may cause a change of behaviour in the abused child, and a pattern of behaviour in the perpetrator. The behaviour in the child will obviously vary a great deal with the age of the child. The child may:

- withdraw from physical contact
- withdraw from close relationships with adults and children
- be apprehensive when other children cry
- be frightened of parents/carers
- fear returning home
- show reluctance for the parents to be contacted
- either refuse to discuss the injury, or may give improbable excuses
- be reluctant to undress for PE or swimming, or to remove clothes in hot weather
- fear medical help or assistance
- display frozen awareness – constant watchfulness of adults' reactions to him or herself
- display self-destructive behaviour
- display aggression towards other children and adults
- have a history of running away
- show a change in eating pattern either by refusing food or over-eating.

If the perpetrator is the parent/carer he or she may:

- keep the child at home for unexplained reasons
- be unwilling to offer explanation for injuries
- give unlikely excuses to explain injuries
- fail to obtain treatment for injuries
- hold extreme views on discipline and control.

Neglect

Neglect is the failure to provide minimum standards of care to meet the basic needs of children.

> **Activity**
> List the needs of children to ensure optimum growth and development. Is it possible to list these in any order of priority?

Neglect can be a very invidious form of maltreatment, which can go on for a long time. It implies the failure of the parents to act properly in safeguarding the health, safety and well-being of the child. It includes nutritional neglect, failure to provide medical care or to protect a child from physical and social danger.

C.H. Kempe

We will look at neglect under three headings, but the three are often interrelated.

PHYSICAL NEGLECT

Signs of physical neglect
The child may be:
- underweight, small for his or her age, with poor muscle tone and a dry wrinkled skin
- constantly hungry, found scavenging for food, displaying an enormous appetite if food is available, emaciated, and may have a distended abdomen
- dirty with his or her personal hygiene needs not being met, and may smell of urine; he or she will appear dirty and uncared for, with unbrushed hair and teeth; and clothing will be dirty and inappropriate for the time of year, possibly too large or too small
- suffering from severe and persistent napkin rash and/or cradle cap
- prone to frequent accidents through lack of supervision
- constantly tired or lethargic
- frequently unwell, with repeated colds and coughs, stomach upsets, and rashes – advice will not be sought for medical problems, and they will remain untreated
- frequently late for school or nursery and overall attendance will be poor.

Behavioural indicators of physical neglect
The child may display:
- low self-esteem and lack of confidence
- neurotic behaviour, such as rocking, hair twisting, head banging, and excessive masturbation
- inability to make social relationships
- destructive and aggressive tendencies
- compulsive stealing, particularly of food
- clinging behaviour to any adult.

EDUCATIONAL NEGLECT

Signs and behavioural indicators of educational neglect
A child who lacks stimulation from his or her home environment will find difficulty in achieving at school or nursery. Take care not to apportion blame to the parents as the neglect may have been unavoidable. For example, children from families fleeing from persecution in their own country may arrive in nurseries and schools with little experience of books, puzzles and games. Educational neglect may be shown by:
- poor language skills
- low self-esteem and lack of confidence
- developmental delay
- short concentration span
- limited experiences
- inattention to a special educational need
- unfamiliarity with books, stories and rhymes

- unfamiliarity with jigsaws and construction toys, unused to any form of creative play
- difficulty in expressing ideas, and understanding new concepts.

Activity

List three ways in which an infant school could help a 5-year-old whose experiences of life outside the family were very limited?

EMOTIONAL NEGLECT

Signs and behavioural indicators of emotional neglect

The parents may withdraw love from the child and fail to provide a home filled with warmth, interest and care. The parents often express unrealistic expectations in the behaviour of the child.

The child may display:

- difficulty in making appropriate relationships with children and adults, and may be clinging or withdrawn
- lack of discrimination in their attachment to an adult, and may be over-friendly to all
- fear of new situations
- inability to express feelings
- extreme comfort habits, such as rocking, using a dummy or masturbating
- low self-esteem, and lack of confidence
- unwillingness to take risks, either physical or intellectual.

In all forms of neglect, the adult may display:

- lack of responsibility, for example continually sending other people to collect the child from nursery or school, continually leaving the child unsupervised
- lack of warmth
- uncaring attitude
- signs of stress
- no interest in the child's progress or activities.

CASE STUDY

Alice is a small girl, aged 2 years and 2 months. She is behind in her developmental progress and is not gaining in weight and height as one would expect. She has been in day care for four months, and is the youngest of four children. Her mother is now a single parent, Alice's father having left home shortly before her birth, with no further contact. She is often collected late, and by different people.

Alice is not an easy child to look after in the group, always demanding attention and is very clinging with adults. She is frightened of new situations. She enjoys her food, and eats well in the nursery, usually asking for second helpings.

- Do you think there is cause for concern? Why?
- What observations might help you to find out more about her situation?
- What records should you maintain for this child and her family?
- How might you improve your communication with the mother?
- Are there any special activities you might devise to help Alice with her social behaviour?

Emotional abuse

Emotional abuse includes a child being continually terrorised, berated, or rejected.

C.H. Kempe

A child who is brought up in a home where there is little or inconsistent love or warmth, will find it difficult to respond appropriately to his or her own or other people's emotional needs. This is even more true of children who are continually and repetitively bullied, made scape-goats and told that they are stupid and a failure or are constantly ridiculed, shouted at and undermined.

SIGNS AND BEHAVIOURAL INDICATORS OF EMOTIONAL ABUSE

A child who is emotionally abused may display:
- fear of new situations
- comfort-seeking behaviour
- speech disorders, such as stammering and stuttering
- all-round developmental delay
- inappropriate emotional responses
- inability to cope with making errors
- extremes of passivity or aggression
- fear of parents being contacted
- low self-esteem and lack of confidence
- self-mutilation, by head-banging, pulling out hair and picking at skin
- poor concentration span
- stealing and telling lies
- wetting and soiling after the age you would expect a child to be clean and dry
- attention-seeking behaviour
- inability to have fun
- poor social relationships
- temper tantrums which are not age-appropriate.

To think about
'Child abuse would be greatly reduced if mothers were discouraged from working outside the home'. Do you agree with this statement?

An adult who is an emotional abuser may:

- show dislike or rejection of the child
- have a history of neglect and abuse themselves
- be locked in conflict with a partner
- be mentally ill
- be abusing drugs or alcohol
- have very unrealistic behavioural or academic expectations of the child
- have a psychopathic personality
- punish harshly, or in a bizarre way
- swing between indulgence and harsh discipline and be unpredictable.

To think about
Policies concerning child abuse need to:
(a) strike a balance between protecting children and respecting family privacy and
(b) be anti-discriminatory and culturally aware.
What difficulties might there be in achieving this?

Sexual abuse

Sexual abuse is:

> . . . *the involvement of dependent developmentally immature children and adolescents in sexual activities that they do not fully comprehend, are unable to give informed consent to and that violate the social taboos of family roles.*
>
> *Schechter and Roberge*

It is a betrayal of trust and responsibility and an abuse of power that allows the perpetrator to coerce a child to take part in sexual activity.

Sexual abuse happens to boys and girls, and is perpetrated by both men and women. It ranges from showing children pornographic material, or touching them inappropriately to penetration, rape and incest. It is found in all cultures and in all classes of society, in all types of families, and across all religious groups. It can start with new-born babies. The majority of children who are abused know the perpetrator, who is often a member of the family, a close friend or someone in a position of trust. Any act committed by a stranger would be considered sexual assault rather than sexual abuse and would be handled by the police and criminal courts. In very young children, because they trust the loved adult, it may take some years before they realise that the abuse does not happen to everyone. They may feel it is wrong, but have no experience to compare it with.

More than any other form of abuse, sexual abuse within the family is a way of displaying power. It rarely involves the use of physical force, as children are trusting and dependent. They want to please and gain love and approval. They believe that adults are always right. The abuse often begins gradually and increases over time. It is a violation of a child's right to a normal healthy trusting relationship and often causes difficulty when the child becomes an adult in making satisfactory sexual relationships.

> **To think about**
> The medical diagnosis of child abuse should never be based on the assessment of just one doctor. Do you agree, and why?

PHYSICAL SIGNS OF SEXUAL ABUSE OR ASSAULT

The child may:
- sustain bruises, scratches or bites to the genital and anal area, chest, neck or abdomen
- have bloodstained or torn underclothing
- show semen on the skin or clothing
- complain of soreness or discomfort in the anal or vaginal areas, or in the throat
- complain of common ailments, such as stomach pains or headaches
- cry hysterically when the napkin or clothing is removed
- display bleeding in the throat, anal or vaginal areas
- experience discomfort when walking or sitting
- experience pain when urinating.

Boys may complain of:
- a swollen penis
- discharge from the penis.

Girls may complain of:
- vaginal discharge.

If referred to a paediatrician, the following may be detected:
- sexually transmitted disease
- semen in the vagina or anus
- internal small cuts in the vagina or anus
- abnormal swelling (dilation) of the vagina or anus
- thrush and urinary tract infections.

BEHAVIOURAL INDICATORS OF SEXUAL ABUSE OR ASSAULT

Quite often, there are no physical indicators of abuse, and the recognition of behavioural indicators becomes crucial.

The child may:
- show fear of a particular person
- regress developmentally
- display insecurity and cling to parents
- behave in a way sexually inappropriate to his or her age, showing an obsession with sexual matters, particularly in doll and role play
- produce drawings of sex organs, such as erect penises and huge breasts
- display withdrawn, sad behaviour and appear unhappy and confused

- demonstrate variations in appetite, perhaps leading to an eating disorder
- demonstrate poor concentration
- show a change in sleeping habits, becoming wakeful or complaining of chronic nightmares
- begin wetting again when previously dry
- act in a placatory or flirtatious way, or in an inappropriately mature way
- be unable to sustain social relationships with other children
- show a range of unpredictable behaviour from withdrawn and fearful to aggressive and hurtful
- introduce obscene words into their language
- display low self-esteem and lack confidence.

Young children will often display many of these behavioural traits at one time or another without them being indicators of sexual abuse. Warning bells should ring if these persist for long periods, or if many of them happen together.

As children develop their language and independence, you may become aware of other behavioural indicators. The child may:

- start to drop hints about secrets
- ask if you can keep secrets
- talk about 'a friend's' problem
- tell lies
- bathe excessively or have poor personal hygiene
- display phobic or panic attacks
- steal or cheat, perhaps in the hope of being caught
- have unexplained amounts of money
- be reluctant to undress for games, swimming or PE
- be reluctant to join in outside activities
- refuse to see or express dislike of certain people
- develop eating disorders, such as anorexia or bulimia
- become severely depressed
- display poor self-image, frequently describing him or herself as dirty, evil or wicked
- attempt to run away from home.

CASE STUDY

Sarah, aged 4 years, has been attending a nursery class for twelve months. One morning she complains of having a sore bottom and when taken to the lavatory the child-care practitioner notices bloodstains on her pants. Sarah says that John, her mother's boyfriend for the past two months, 'pokes' her bottom. She says she does not like John as he gets angry if she is unwilling to 'play the game'.

- Do you think Sarah is being abused? What type or types of abuse?
- What other indicators would you look for?
- What might be the likely physical, emotional and educational effects on a child in the short-term and in the long-term?
- What are Sarah's immediate needs in this situation?
- What are the needs of the family?

Failure to thrive

Children who are abused are often diagnosed as 'failing to thrive'. This refers to children who fail to grow in the expected way, for no organic or genetic reason. It is important to rule out organic factors such as malabsorption of nutrients, infection and major illness. Other children will fail to thrive because of stress, poverty, or poor parenting. The latter may be linked with neglect, but need not be deliberate. All children who fail to thrive should be referred to a paediatrician. Percentile charts will be used to assess and monitor the child's growth, head circumference and height, in addition to other investigations. Further information about the use of percentile charts is contained in Appendix 2. It is important to obtain a clear medical history of the child.

Children who are failing to thrive because of abuse or neglect, will often start to gain weight and grow if removed from the family home for a period of time.

> **Activity**
> Joanne Brown aged 2½ years, and her sister Sally aged 6 months have just been admitted to your day nursery on the recommendation of their health visitor. Joanne has 'failed to thrive' and is being seen by the paediatrician at the local hospital. When you lift Sally out of the pram you notice maggots crawling under the mattress.
> 1 What is your immediate course of action?
> 2 How might you help the children in the long-term?
> 3 What agencies would be involved in supporting this family?

Organised abuse

The physical signs and behavioural indicators have already been described under sexual and emotional abuse. This type of abuse is often associated with bizarre sadistic behaviour, arousing extreme terror in the victims. The existence of this type of abuse is often debated, but the fear of the victims makes disclosure very difficult and thus it is often impossible to collect objective evidence.

Munchausen syndome by proxy (sometimes known as Meadows syndrome)

This is a rare and severe personality disorder, usually found in women, who create the symptoms of fictitious disease in the child. It usually involves mothers who are very closely bonded to their children, and who tend to have detailed medical knowledge. The symptoms are real and convincing: they may range from putting blood on a child's napkin or into a urine sample, to giving laxatives to cause diarrhoea. This may be followed by inappropriate and painful tests in hospital, or even submitting the child to an operation.

There have even been cases where dangerous drugs or poisonous substances have been administered to the child, while the child was under observation in hospital. It is difficult to diagnose the condition, as often the mother is very attentive and concerned, and may form close relationships with the hospital staff.

Child-care practitioners should be concerned if a seemingly healthy child is being constantly admitted to hospital.

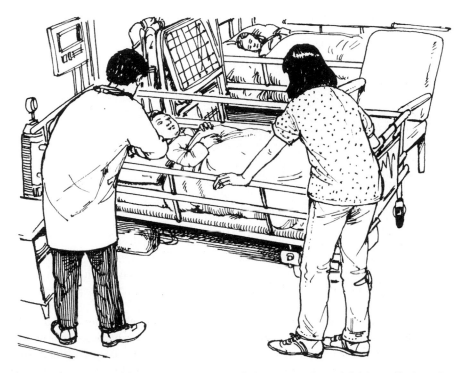

A woman who creates the symptoms of disease in her child is suffering from Munchausen syndrome by proxy

GOOD PRACTICE

Develop good practice in recognising abuse.
1 Be alert to all signs of abuse, but be careful not to jump to conclusions: many of the signs can be put down to other causes.
2 Keep up to date and have a good knowledge of developmental· norms and age-appropriate behaviour.
3 Remember that abuse occurs in all strata of society and in all cultures and religions.

4 If you suspect abuse, be discreet, and discuss your suspicions only with your line manager.

5 Your role is to observe, record and report suspected abuse, not to investigate it.

6 Be very tactful and sensitive in your handling of and communication with a child whom you suspect has been abused.

7 Remember that an abused child generally will have experienced more than one kind of abuse.

8 Do not question the child again once disclosure has taken place, as you may influence legal proceedings and increase the child's anxiety and distress.

Female sexual abusers

During the nineties there has been a growing awareness that men are not the only sexual abusers of young children. Michele Elliott, the Director of Kidscape, wrote in an article, 'Social work today', 12.03.92, after taking part in a local radio phone-in programme where the issue was first raised, that one hundred people contacted her stating that they had been abused by a female, frequently acting alone and not under the influence of a male partner.

There are few statistics showing how much sexual abuse is perpetrated by women. This may be because:

■ the concept of women as abusers is threatening, as women are perceived as nurturing caregivers, the natural protectors of children

■ women are not supposed to be sexually aggressive

■ people who have disclosed have not been believed and have been told that they are fantasising

■ people find it difficult to understand that women could sexually abuse a child.

Twenty years ago, sexual abuse of young children by either sex was thought to be extremely rare. However, the media and Childline have together raised the awareness of the general public, and it might have to be accepted that sexual abuse by females is more prevalent than previously thought.

Activity
Women appear to have become more assertive and aggressive during the last decade. Identify positive and negative effects of this development.

You, as child-care practitioners, are in daily contact with young children, have developed sensitive and accurate observation skills, and have a sound knowledge of children's developmental progress. This makes you the professional most likely to recognise signs and behavioural indicators of abuse.

KEY TERMS

You need to know what these words and phrases mean. Go back through the chapter and make sure that you understand:

accidental injury
behavioural indicators
development of the whole child
developmental delay
female sexual abusers
fingertip bruising
frozen awareness

inflicted injury
informed consent
low self-esteem
percentile charts
perpetrator
sexual assault
social taboos

Resources

Elliott, M., 'The ultimate taboo' in *Nursery World*: 2.11.95; *Female Sexual Abuse of Children: the Ultimate Taboo*, Pitman, 1996

Horwath, J. and Lawson, B. (Eds), *Trust Betrayed: Munchausen Syndrome by Proxy*, National Children's Bureau, 1995

Neale, B., Bools, C. and Meadow, R., 'Problems in the assessment and management of Munchausen syndrome by proxy abuse' in *Children and Society*, Vol. 5,1991

O'Hagan, K., *Emotional and Psychological Abuse of Children*, OUP, 1993

Wallace, W., 'Duty of care' in *Nursery World*: 24.10.96

5 FOLLOWING RECOGNITION OF ABUSE

> **This chapter covers:**
> - **Building relationships**
> - **Protecting the child in the home setting**
> - **Policies and procedures in an establishment**
> - **Observations and record-keeping**
> - **Referrals**
> - **Child protection conferences**
> - **Abuse in the workplace**
> - **Resources**

One of the first things that you will do, when you enter employment, is to find out the policies and procedures that dictate the practice of the workplace. This should include procedures to be followed if you suspect a child is in need of protection.

Building relationships

Unless there are obvious physical signs of abuse, you probably would not be aware that a child was in need of protection, unless you knew the children in your care very well and had built up good relationships with them. Children are often reluctant to reveal any unhappiness at home, and young children do not have the experience to compare their home life with that of others. Once you get to know the child and the family and have established a trusting relationship, the child may hint at an unhappy home life. Occasionally your suspicions may be aroused by the parents/carers who may display a lack of self-control.

Trusting your intuition is not good enough for a professional child-care worker. Having informed your line manager or designated teacher of your concerns, you should observe the child closely, and record changes in behaviour, precocious language, or expressions of unmet needs, so that you are armed with some objective evidence. You may, at this stage, decide to talk to the child's parents/carers, tactfully seeking an explanation for an injury or a change in the behaviour of the child. You may wish to record the parents'/carers' responses. At this stage, it might be useful to seek advice from your local child protection adviser from the social services department.

> **Activity**
> Refer to the case study of Tracey on page 65. You have made the decision to discuss Tracey's injuries with her mother. How do you see yourself conducting this interview? Role play the interview with a colleague in your group.

Protecting the child in the home setting

WORKING AS A NANNY

If you are working in a family as a nanny, and you suspect abuse, it is often difficult to find someone with whom to discuss your suspicions. Belonging to a union is useful in this case, as they would advise you on how to proceed. If you have recently left college, your tutor may be willing to listen to you, and help you judge the situation. Observe the child or children closely, and keep a record of any odd behaviour.

Remember that some families will bring up their children in a way you might feel is bizarre and very different from the way you might have been brought up. They might think that the human body is nothing to be ashamed of, and both adults and children may walk around the house with no clothes on. You might be able to talk about this with the parents if you find it embarrassing. Be careful not to be judgemental or jump to conclusions. It is sensible, before you enter employment, to discuss the parents' attitude to discipline and control. If this is very different from your own views and your understanding of good practice it might be wise to seek a different post.

If you actually witness abuse of any sort you cannot ignore it. Your first duty is to protect the child. If the abuse is emotional or educational, you should try to discuss this with the parents, pointing out the effects on the child and attempting to use your knowledge and skills to show how such abuse would have a later detrimental effect.

If the abuse results in physical injury or sexual exploitation you should refer to social services or get in touch with your health visitor, the NSPCC, or the police. You should not feel disloyal in doing this. You might find it helpful to contact your union to advise and support you in this matter. You should certainly inform the agency that found you the position.

Be very sure of the facts before taking any action. Obviously, taking any matters like this into the public arena may result in you losing your job, and you may even face litigation.

WORKING AS A CHILDMINDER

If you are looking after other people's children as a childminder, you will be registered and inspected by social services. If you have some unsubstantiated concerns about a child, you may wish to discuss it with your health visitor or day-care advisor. If you suspect that one of the children in your charge may be suffering from abuse, you have a responsibility to report it at once to the Social Services Department

Activity
What routine records might you be advised to keep when working as a childminder?

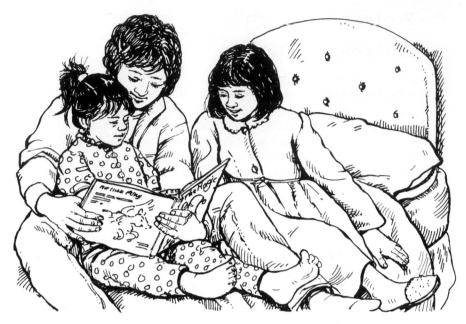

Nannies must be alert to protecting the children in their care

Policies and procedures in an establishment

If you feel concerned about a child, the first thing you should do is look again at the procedures outlining the lines of responsibility. See page 81 for an example of a child protection policy document. The procedures adopted in any institution should coincide with the procedures outlined by the Area Child Protection Committee (ACPC). A similar document should also be available within your establishment.

Observations and record-keeping

If you notice any physical signs of abuse, for example bruises or burns that are revealed during PE or rest sessions, or when changing a napkin, you must make a written, dated and timed note of the facts immediately, as, if they are not written within twenty-four hours they are not legally admissible. It would be advisable to ask another professional adult to confirm your findings discreetly. It should then be reported at once to your manager or designated teacher being careful not to draw unnecessary attention to the child or making the child feel uncomfortable.

All staff need to use similar methods of recording and share the responsibility for this. In some establishments diagrams of children's bodies may be available to help you record locations and patterns of injuries accurately.

CHILD PROTECTION POLICY

OBJECTIVE

To ensure staff maintain vigilance to enable them to spot signs or symptoms associated with child abuse, and inform relevant Statutory authorities. To ensure staff and regular volunteers have been vetted for previous relevant convictions which may make them unacceptable for caring for children.

PROCEDURE

Staff should be aware of a change in a child's behaviour or appearance, and react accordingly. This is especially relevant in the case of young babies who are unable to tell you if any abuse has taken place. This may necessitate having a confidential discussion with other members of the staff team and they may have some useful observations to share. At these discussions it would be decided whether it was necessary to monitor the situation for a few days or weeks, or whether to take immediate action. The Co-ordinator, in dicussion with Head Office is responsible for contacting the Social Services if there is reason to believe that child abuse is taking place.

Some signs or symptoms may have a reasonable explanation e.g. extensive bruising may occur because the child is a haemophiliac (information such as this should be noted on the child's Information Consent Form).

Staff must be prepared to listen carefully and sympathetically to any children who wish to confide in them, and to take them seriously. It is rare for young children to make false accusations, especially of sexual abuse, and it must always be investigated. ***Under no circumstances should an adult ask a child questions.***

Staff must record everything that has been noticed and any decisions/actions taken. Everything that has been said by the child must be recorded exactly.

Children must not feel that they are being interviewed by staff.

Information must be kept confidentially.

Example of a child protection policy document

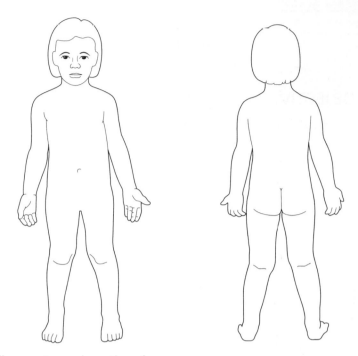

Blank diagram to use in noting abuse

You may ask the child about the injury, if he or she can communicate with language. Keep it brief and open-ended saying, for example, 'What a nasty burn on your arm! Can you remember how you got it?' Record the child's answer and general response. Do not probe any further or push for an explanation, as this may distress the child.

Where there are no physical signs of abuse and the issue is less clear cut, but nonetheless you feel uneasy about the way a child has started to behave, it is sensible to keep a diary over a period of time. Note any incidents, accidents or problems that the child has experienced, record any anxieties or fears that the child confides to you, and note carefully any absences, especially if these are for a week or more. These records should be dated and completely factual, containing no hearsay or opinions, and completed within twenty-four hours. See page 84 for an example of a completed record sheet. Inform your line manager that you are keeping these records. Remember that parents are entitled to see these records and observations if they so wish. If there has been abuse, you will be asked to produce your written notes at a child protection conference or even in court.

Activity
You are working in a day-care setting and a 4-year-old whispers that his 'uncle' had touched him somewhere that he did not like.

How would you feel? How would you respond to the child? What might you do?

ANYWHERE NURSERY

Name   Date of birth   Start date   Class/group

Date Time	Incident	Physical injury	Non attendance	Conversation	Behaviour causing concern	Action	Signature

Example of a record sheet

ANYWHERE NURSERY

Name Jane Smith Date of birth 10.3.94 Start date 8.9.97 Class/group Nursery

Date Time	Incident	Physical injury	Non attendance	Conversation	Behaviour causing concern	Action	Signature
30.9.97 10 am		Bruises seen on both arms		Child states she fell off bike		Chart started	CAH
9.10.97 9.30 am 12.15 pm	Child very hungry asked for food at 9.30 am Had 3 helpings at lunch					noted	CAH
15.10.97 -26.10.97			F.T.A	Mother states child unwell Did not see G.P.		Discussed with Line Manager	CAH JF
29.10.97 all day				Avoids contact with adults & peers	Quiet, withdrawn passive	Observations to be made over next week	CAH
16.11.97 3.30 pm	Mother collects child, smells of drink					Discussed with Line Manager	CAH
17.11.97 11 am		?small burns on legs		No response from child	Crying in home corner	Discussed with Line Manager Designated teacher involved	CAH
17.11.97			F.T.A			To contact Social Services	JF

Example of a completed record sheet

Referrals

If you are working in the home setting, and have been unable to communicate with the parents, you might have to refer a child directly to social services, the family health visitor, or the NSPCC. Persevere if the telephone seems to be permanently engaged. In an emergency situation you may have to go directly to the police.

While working in an establishment, it would be unlikely to be your direct responsibility to refer the child, but you must act promptly in informing your line manager, following the procedures set down.

If no action is taken, and you feel very sure that the child is in need of protection, you may have to take direct action yourself, even though this might make things very awkward for you. First try to seek the permission of your manager to arrange a consultation with the social services department. If this is denied, you will have to proceed on your own initiative. This will be a rare situation, but you would have to face up to it. Remember that the Children Act, 1989, states that 'the welfare of the child is paramount'. You are professionally responsible for your practice and actions. If your manager is not treating your concerns seriously you might proceed by speaking directly to someone who has specialist knowledge of child protection procedures.

If a child urgently requires medical treatment, an ambulance should be called and the child taken to the local accident and emergency department. Under no circumstances drive the child there in your car. If you suspect that the injury is non-accidental inform the Duty Officer at the Social Services Department. Contact the parents/carers immediately, informing them of the specific injury or symptoms, but do not discuss your suspicions of abuse at this time.

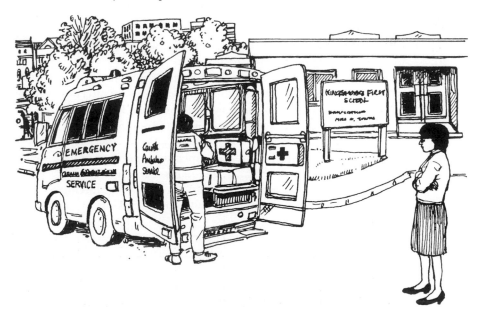

Call an ambulance if urgent medical treatment is required

Child protection conferences

Once a child has been referred and the matter investigated, a child protection conference may be called. This is where your carefully kept records and observations will be most useful to all the agencies involved. You have a key role at these conferences, as you will have had regular daily contact with the child and the family, and have established a warm and trusting relationship that has facilitated communication. Your line manager may accompany you to the conference and this may help you to ensure that your voice is heard. He or she might have a contribution to make in reporting concerns raised by other members of the staff team.

Prepare your contribution in advance, always being factual and objective. You may wish to take your observations, a diary, account of conversations, and a short written report summarising your concerns. Remember parents have a right to attend conferences. This might make you feel uncomfortable, but the presence of the parents is in the interest of the child.

If the child is placed on a register and a protection plan is drawn up at the conference, you should be clear about the role you and your establishment will play. You may have some suggestions to make based on your knowledge of the child. Your presence at the case conference will help to ensure that the discussion remains child-centred, as many of the other agencies will be more familiar with the needs of the parents, rather than the child.

The review dates set at the conference may require you to provide written reports on the progress of the child and the family.

Abuse in the workplace

If you suspect one of your colleagues of child abuse, you will have to act on your suspicions. The abuse may take the form of:

- *emotional abuse*, such as shouting at children, frightening children with terrifying stories, threatening to punish children, withdrawing affection, isolating a child to sit on a 'naughty chair' or stand in the corner, forcing children to give affection when they do not want to, taunting children in a sarcastic manner, or racial abuse
- *neglect*, such as leaving children unsupervised, not providing a stimulating and safe environment, or not changing napkins regularly
- *physical abuse*, such as smacking a child, force-feeding, forcing a child to remain on a potty or the lavatory for a long time, shaking or pushing a child, or restraining a child roughly
- *sexual abuse*, such as touching children inappropriately, taking a suspiciously long time in the bathroom area when supervising children, making opportunities for time alone with children without a specific, known purpose, or inappropriate conversations with children.

If you feel that there is cause for alarm, you should keep a record of all worrying behaviour, noting dates, places and times, children involved, conversations and language, and children's response to such behaviour. These observations should be kept to yourself until such time as you have collated enough data to discuss the situation with your line manager. There are procedures to follow, and you may well be involved in contributing to disciplinary procedures. Whistle blowers are never popular, but you have to put the needs of the children before your own. Your union may be in a position to advise and support you.

Activity
Identify the range of feelings you might have when challenging the practice of a colleague.

Obviously there are degrees of aberrant behaviour and if your colleague behaves in a satisfactory manner in most areas of the work but, for example, insisted on standing children in a corner, you could perhaps discuss this, pointing out that it is not good practice to isolate children in this manner. If there is no change in behaviour, you might decide to bring up the matter of suitable discipline at a staff meeting.

Activity
What areas of behaviour would you consider serious enough to report a colleague to his or her line manager? What areas would you feel you might be able to deal with yourself?

PROTECT YOURSELF

When working in any child-care setting, you need to be aware that you are in a vulnerable situation. Remarks made by very young children can be misconstrued. The media have made sure that any institutional abuse has been brought to the public's attention, and while this is quite right, it nevertheless makes working in the public domain an area where one's behaviour has to be professional at all times, and open to scrutiny.

There are steps you can take to prevent being unjustly accused of abuse.

- Make sure your record keeping is up to date. Registers, observations, records of achievement, accident and incident report forms etc. should all be written up daily and kept in a safe place. If an accident occurs, ensure that it is recorded and that this is witnessed by another member of staff.
- If you are suspicious or concerned about any child or colleague, report these concerns to your line manager and keep a written record.
- Attend staff meetings and local staff support groups.
- Belong to a union or professional association.
- Keep the child's parent/carer and your line manager informed of any incidents, accidents or events that have occurred during the day.

- Ensure that children are well supervised and do not leave them in the care of unauthorised people.
- If a child behaves in a sexually inappropriate manner towards you, record the incident, and make sure that another adult knows about it. Some young children like to kiss adults on the mouth. You should discourage this, and if it persists, record it and discuss it with a colleague.

As a student you would not perform any intimate task, such as changing a napkin or wiping bottoms without a member of staff there, and in the same way, it is wise to make sure someone else is present when you first start work at an establishment. With a new child, it may be possible to encourage the mother to stay and carry out these tasks until a good relationship is firmly established. Encourage independence in children and do not carry out any intimate tasks that they are quite capable of doing for themselves.

Children need affectionate and warm relationships and you should attempt to meet their needs, but if a child tells you that you are doing something that they do not like, stop at once. Take time to build up relationships. Avoid spending excessive amounts of time alone with any one child. See below for a summary on how to protect yourself from suspicion of child abuse in the placement.

HOW TO PROTECT YOURSELF FROM SUSPICION OF CHILD ABUSE IN THE PLACEMENT

1 Do not show favouritism or spend too long with one child, unless it is following an observation and with the approval of your Supervisor.

2 Do not take children to the lavatory by themselves until you have settled in placement, and are aware of the policy of the Nursery.

3 Carry out intimate tasks for children in the presence of other staff.

4 Do not arrange to see children or their families outside placement on any pretext. Do not agree to any baby sitting arrangements.

5 Keep a daily log/diary to record your activities and movements.

6 Use appropriate language in front of all the children

7 Be circumspect in how you approach children, do not touch or pick up a child who does not want to be touched or picked up.

8 Touches from children that worry you should be reported at once to your Supervisor, as well as any other incidents that make you uncomfortable.

9 Do not ask children to keep secrets.

10 Managing children's challenging behaviour should never involve handling a child roughly.

11 Do not shout at or use a sarcastic approach with children.

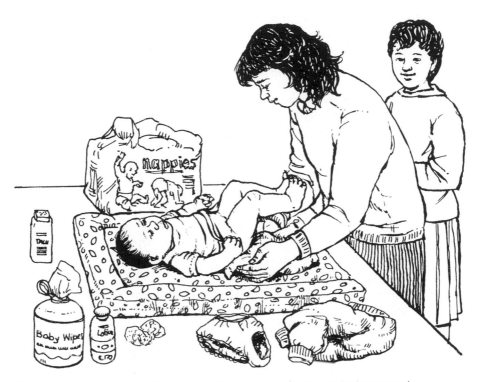

Make sure someone else is present when you perform any intimate task

If, in spite of all your care, a complaint has been made against you, you will obviously experience feelings of distress and anxiety, but do not panic. All complaints have to be investigated. This is a legal requirement and everyone involved will be trying to reach an objective decision. Keep a record of all conversations you have, both face-to-face and on the telephone, concerning this matter. Include times, dates, places and participants. Keep copies of all correspondence. You may wish to seek legal advice, either independently or through your union or professional association. A senior member of staff should advise you of internal procedures.

Once the matter has been resolved, and you are found to be blameless, you may find it useful to discuss the matter with your line or senior manager to prevent such a distressing reoccurrence. You might find it helpful to seek post-traumatic stress counselling. Your managers or your professional association might be able to help you with this.

Recognition of abuse is always followed by specific procedures that have to be adhered to, even though this may result in a stressful and uncomfortable workplace environment. This may be particularly difficult to cope with if you have experienced abuse yourself. Nevertheless, as you fully understand as a professional person, the child has to be protected.

Resources

Bond, H., 'Emotional abuse' in *Nursery World*: 4.8.94

Cloke, C. and Naish, J., *Key Issues in Child Protection for Health Visitors and Nurses*, NSPCC and Longman, 1992

Hobart, C. and Frankel, J., *A Practical Guide to Child Observation*, Stanley Thornes (Publishers) Ltd 1994

Hobbs, C.J. and Wynne, J.M., *Balliere's Clinical Paediatrics: Child Abuse*, Balliere, Tindall, 1993

National Children's Bureau Highlight, *Child Sexual Abuse, Highlight No. 119,* 1993

National Early Years Network, *Recognising Child Abuse*, (booklet)

Neale, B., Bools, C. and Meadow, R., 'Problems in the assessment and management of Muchausen syndrome by proxy abuse' in *Children and Society*, Vol.5, 1991

Woolfson, R., 'Munchausen syndrome by proxy – the mysterious syndrome' in *Nursery World*: 15.6.89

6 ROLES OF THE DIFFERENT AGENCIES IN PROTECTING CHILDREN

> **This chapter covers:**
> - The role of social services
> - The role of the health service
> - The role of the education service
> - The role of the legal system
> - The role of voluntary groups
> - The role of the child-care practitioner
> - Male child-care practitioners
> - Resources

If you are working with children who have been abused, or who are thought to be at risk, you will find yourself working as part of a multi-disciplinary team, which will include representatives from social services, education, the health service and the legal system, and possibly other voluntary groups or organisations such as the NSPCC, the Family Rights Group (FRG) and Parents Against Injustice (PAIN). Each group that you work with will have received different training, and may have a different perspective on child protection. A great deal of hard work has to be done to make these disparate groups act together in harmony in the interests of the child. It is important to note that the only agencies with a duty to investigate, and the power to protect and, if necessary, remove children, are social services departments, the police, and the NSPCC. None of the other agencies have statutory duties or powers to investigate, but play a role as described in local child protection procedures.

> **To think about**
> Children would be better protected if there was a single agency in charge rather than a process of getting disparate groups to work together. Do you agree with this statement? What problems might a single agency face?

The role of social services

THE SOCIAL WORKER

Most social workers, but not all, will hold the Certificate of Qualification in Social Work (CQSW), or the newer Diploma in Social Work (DipSW). These involve courses of study of between two and four years, and include college-based academic study and work-based placements. Recent research (Stone 1990; Scrine 1991) shows that some students had little or no class teaching on child protection. Specific training is usually given after qualification. The social worker works in office-based teams supervised by a team leader. The majority of social workers involved in child protection are female.

Once social services is alerted to potential abuse, usually by a member of another profession though sometimes by a member of the public, the case is allocated to a social worker. The first step is to check records and information held by all concerned agencies: health, education, police, probation and social services. This is to build up as complete a picture as possible of the child and the family, even though it may delay the investigation. The social worker will then interview the person who made the referral, as well as the child, the parents, siblings, and any other relevant person. The social worker's difficult task is to protect the child while building a relationship of trust with the family. It may be necessary for the child to be medically examined. In extreme cases, the social worker may immediately apply to the court for an Emergency Protection Order (EPO), and find a suitable placement in foster or residential care. A child protection conference will be convened and the social worker is responsible for reporting back on the investigation to all agencies concerned before, during and after the conference.

Consistent with the welfare and protection of children procedures the social worker must keep the parents fully informed, enabling them to share concerns about their children's welfare, attempting to involve parents in planning and decision making, and showing respect and consideration for their opinions.

The social worker will be continually involved with the family and will be responsible for the continuing assessment and review of the situation and will be in

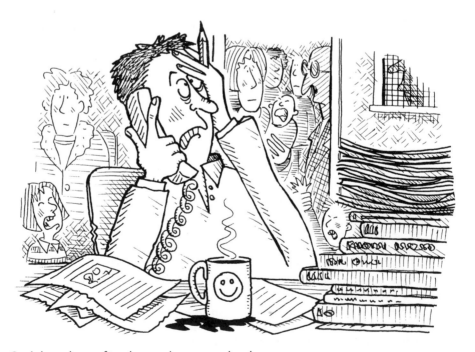

Social workers often have a large case load

frequent contact with all members of the multi-disciplinary team. The formal end of the investigation may, quite often, mean the start of long-term work with the family.

The public demands a great deal from social workers, who do not always have the power to implement decisions, and who very often have a large case load which makes it difficult for them to follow through each case with the thoroughness child protection demands.

THE SOCIAL WORK MANAGER

A social work manager will always be a trained social worker. Some social work managers may hold a management qualification. All will be experienced in child protection work. The conduct of a case is the responsibility of the social work manager, and he or she will be involved in the supervision and monitoring of the social worker, from the investigation phase through to the long-term plans for the child.

THE FOSTER CARER

There is no qualification requirement to become a foster carer, but there has been an increase in training in some authorities. A foster carer is assessed, registered, and supported by a social worker and gives a home to children who need care away from their own families, either long-term or for a short stay. Some of these children will have been abused. The Children Act 1989 expects the foster carer to be more aware of children's cultural and religious needs and to play a more active role in working with the natural parents of the children in their care.

The role of the health service

THE PAEDIATRICIAN

A paediatrician is a qualified medical doctor who has undertaken specialist training in child health and further training in child protection. Paediatricians played a key role in bringing child abuse to the attention of the public in the sixties and seventies. The paediatrician works in the community, promoting health and assessing development, and in hospitals working with ill children, and has a central role in diagnosing physical abuse, and also neglect, 'failure to thrive' and sexual abuse.

Historically, paediatricians have been regarded as powerful, and it has been difficult to challenge their diagnoses. The Cleveland inquiry questioned their infallibility. The paediatrician has a key role in the organisation of the area child protection committees. He or she can make arrangements for children to be admitted to hospital for assessment, and will be involved in interviewing parents. He or she may be required to give written reports that may be used in legal proceedings and is sometimes required to attend court to present evidence.

THE HEALTH VISITOR

A health visitor is a trained nurse with a one-year specialist training in health visiting, including issues concerning child protection. Many health visitors are also midwives. Working primarily with pre-school children and their families the health visitor visits all families in a specific location or who are attached to a general practice. He or she will undertake intensive visiting to those children who are at risk of abuse, working closely with a social worker and in partnership with the parents.

THE GENERAL PRACTITIONER

A General Practitioner (GP) is a qualified medical doctor who has undertaken further GP training. One aspect of this training will be paediatrics, and child protection will be included. The GP is responsible for primary health care of the families on his or her caseload. Despite the often excellent knowledge GPs have of the families, they tend not to play a significant central role in child protection cases, frequently finding it difficult to attend child protection conferences and liaise with other professions. This is unfortunate as the GP is often the first to become aware of indications of child abuse and neglect.

To think about
What reasons might there be for the GP not wishing or being unable to become too involved in child protection cases?

THE CHILD PSYCHIATRIST

The child psychiatrist is a qualified doctor with substantial further psychiatric training. He or she is not involved in all areas of child protection but may be involved in assessments of individual children and their families. Where appropriate, the child psychiatrist may be asked to contribute to multi-disciplinary team work, and his or her evidence is highly regarded in cases that come to court.

THE POLICE SURGEON

The police surgeon is a qualified doctor, and frequently a qualified GP, who has a central role in examining children and obtaining forensic evidence for any legal procedures. A key factor concerning the regard in which some police surgeons are held is the degree of sensitivity they have in their examination of the child and their understanding that they might be the first ones to help the child come to terms with the abuse.

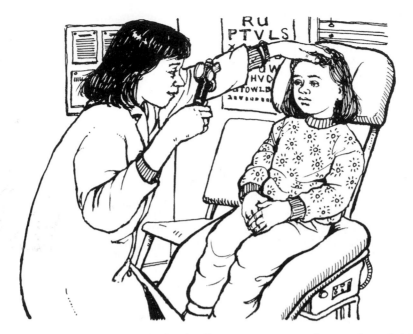

The police surgeon might be the first person to examine an abused child

The role of the education service

After the time spent with their families, children spend most time at school in contact with a range of people who work in the school: headteachers, teachers, child-care practitioners, primary school helpers, dinner ladies, and the school nurse. The child might choose to disclose abuse to any one of these people to whom he or she may feel a special empathy. People who work in a school are in a key position to pick up signs of abuse, and no one more so than child-care practitioners based on their excellent knowledge of child development and normal behaviour and their observational skills.

Since the Children Act 1989 the government has published codes of practice to be implemented in all schools.

- The Local Education Authority (LEA) is required to appoint an official to act as the departmental child protection co-ordinator.
- Schools should be notified by social services of any child who is on the child protection register. This helps them to be alert to the child's pattern of attendance, behaviour and all round development.
- A teacher must be appointed in every school (the designated teacher) to act as a link with the social services department. This is often the headteacher. The LEA is required to keep registers of named staff taking on this role and provide regular training and support.

- All schools must have a written policy outlining procedures and lines of reporting to social services.
- LEA and ACPC procedures should be followed by all branches of the education service.
- Schools are encouraged to develop curriculum plans which help children to develop skills and practices which protect them from abuse, helping them to challenge or speak about distressing situations.

THE HEADTEACHER

The headteacher's approach to child protection may be critical in determining the school's attitude towards the issue, but all educators should be aware that their own behaviour in the classroom should be non-threatening, non-violent and non-judgemental, teaching children to resolve conflict through negotiation and discussion. Young children of both genders are taught caring skills in their play with dolls and in domestic play. Educators should be aware that these skills need to be taught throughout childhood and adolescence, culminating in teaching for parenthood.

THE SCHOOL NURSE

The school nurse has access to information about school children and their families and is concerned with health promotion and monitoring development. He or she has a duty to report suspected abuse, visits most schools regularly, and may be permanently attached to a special school.

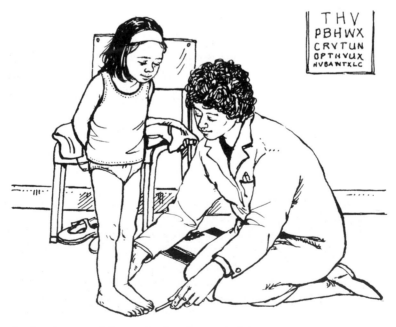

A school nurse visits most schools regularly

THE EDUCATIONAL SOCIAL WORKER

The educational social worker is often the link between the school and the community. He or she is in a good position to recognise abuse within the family and to act as an advisor to the school.

THE EDUCATIONAL PSYCHOLOGIST

The educational psychologist is employed by the psychological services department of the LEA. He or she may be involved in child protection conferences but often his or her role may be after the abuse has been disclosed, when he or she would help the child in educational and therapeutic contexts.

The role of the legal system

The structure of the courts system is shown on page 98.

THE JUDGE

A judge is a qualified barrister who through experience and recommendation has been promoted to the judiciary. He or she will make legal decisions about the most

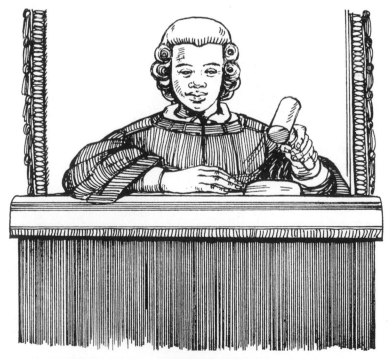

A judge rules on child protection cases heard in court

COURTS

Family Proceedings Court

These magistrates courts, where all care proceedings from the local authority start, deal with simple cases: care and supervision orders, emergency orders, adoption and maintenance and domestic violence.

County Court

These deal with civil matters only. Some county courts have the authority to deal with cases involving children. Judges and other court staff have specialist training. Complicated cases are moved up from the family proceedings court and heard before a judge.

High Court – Family Division

These deal with complicated cases involving difficult legal issues. They will hear any appeal against a judgement from the family proceedings courts.

Court of Appeal

These will hear appeals against decisions of the High Court.

The House of Lords

This is the Court of Final Appeal.

Proceedings

The child's welfare and future life is the priority of the court. All civil court proceedings concerning child protection are confidential and held in a closed court. The courts will decide whether or not to grant an order and what is in the best interests of the child. Blame is not apportioned – that is the responsibility of the criminal courts at another time if appropriate.

Criminal proceedings

Criminal proceedings are entirely separate from care proceedings.

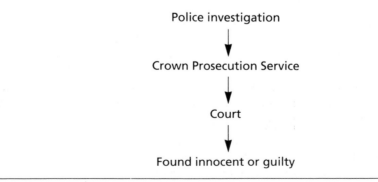

Police investigation

↓

Crown Prosecution Service

↓

Court

↓

Found innocent or guilty

The structure of the courts system

difficult child protection cases referred from the lower courts. The judge may have had some training in child protection procedures. Judges who sit in the Family Division Court will have received intensive training in child protection issues. There are some senior women judges with an excellent understanding of the issues. All judges are extremely well trained and qualified to interpret the law.

THE MAGISTRATE

Few magistrates have any formal legal training or qualification. The magistrate is an amateur, reflecting the views and values of the community. He or she may hold many different qualifications from many areas of work. Some will sit in the Family Proceedings Court to hear public and private cases concerning children. He or she will process the vast majority of cases that come to court, with only about 15 per cent going to a higher court. The magistrate has to receive some specialist training and have experience in dealing with family matters, before he or she can be nominated to sit.

THE COURT CLERK

The clerk functions as the professional legal adviser to the magistrate. He or she will usually have qualified as a solicitor or barrister. During emergency and care proceedings the clerk plays a critical role in controlling legal activity and, being the facilitator and adviser to the magistrate, who is an amateur, has a great deal of power.

THE BARRISTER

If any proceedings concerning child protection reach the County Court or High Court, a barrister will be used to present to the court the case of the local authority or the parents or the child, or any other person involved in the proceedings. The barrister is often involved in chairing independent reviews or inquiries into child deaths or failures in the child protection system. He or she has little specific training in child abuse but may have developed a specialist practice in child protection work.

THE SOLICITOR

The solicitor represents any of the people involved in proceedings in the lower court, and will instruct the barrister on behalf of clients in the higher courts. The local authority will often use a solicitor from its own legal department. The solicitor will be involved in giving advice from an early stage of the process. The Law Society's Children's Panel involves solicitors whose experience has led to a particular skill in this area. Before inclusion in the panel, a solicitor is required to undertake some training in child law and child protection issues.

Activity
Visit a court and recognise the roles of the people in the legal system.

THE POLICE FORCE

The police have a dual role. On the one hand, they are required to investigate whether any criminal law has been broken, and prepare evidence for the court. On the other hand, police involvement is used to protect children at risk, always keeping the best interests of the child in the forefront of their actions. They are likely to be involved in investigating serious physical abuse and all cases of sexual abuse. In this area they will be especially trained to work with social workers in interviewing children to gather and assess evidence of abuse. They are empowered to inform other professionals if an adult has a record of serious crime against children. They are also empowered to help social workers enforce orders under the civil law. The Police and Criminal Evidence Act (1984) gives the police the common law power to enter and search any premises for the purposes of 'saving life or limb'. Exercising of this power could be followed by reception of the child into police protection.

In many areas the police have become very active participants of the area committees for the protection of children. After qualifying as police officers, some may choose to undertake training in this area of work. Many who do so are women, who volunteer for this specialist area of family violence and abuse. Many police forces have developed their own specialist teams.

To think about

Is going to prison the most effective course of action for a perpetrator of abuse? What alternatives might there be?

THE PROBATION OFFICER

The probation officer is a social worker who has completed a specialist option within the course, and is sponsored by the Home Office. His or her role is to serve the legal system by advising the court on child and family matters and to represent the best interests of the alleged offender within the legal process. Like any other professional involved with a family, he or she is required to be observant and to refer and discuss possible abuse within the multi-disciplinary team and if concerned about the safety of a child who lives in the same household as an offender, must inform social services. Over the last twenty years, the probation officer has developed a role in working on the treatment of perpetrators of child sexual abuse, often involving community treatment programmes.

To think about

Professional people such as doctors, lawyers and priests should be prepared to share information about child abuse with other professionals. Does this break the rules of confidentiality?

THE GUARDIAN *AD LITEM*

The guardian *ad litem* (GAL) is always a qualified social worker, well experienced in child protection work, who will have received additional training before undertaking this role. Employed by the local authority or by a voluntary social work organisation as an independent adviser to the court on the needs and best interests of the child the GAL can speak on behalf of the child, and will help the child come to some understanding of the decisions being taken. Often involved in the process from an early stage, such as the first or second interim hearing he or she will investigate and comment upon the original abuse, the child's relationship with the family, rehabilitation, and plans for the future. The GAL does not have any statutory power, but because of his or her independence and experience, exercises considerable influence in the child protection process.

THE OFFICIAL SOLICITOR

The official solicitor will be appointed to cases that start and are completed in the High Court, or which are allocated to the High Court from a lower court, often in cases where there are wider, complex issues or matters of public policy. The official solicitor may act as guardian *ad litem*, but will not be a member of any panel of guardians *ad litem*. They have excellent access to specialists, such as paediatricians and psychiatrists nation-wide.

To think about

All professionals working in child protection should receive more training in racial and cultural aspects of child rearing and modes of discipline.

Knowing that in some cultures corporal punishment is seen to be the norm, how would you react to a child from such a culture being hit with a strap as a form of discipline?

The role of voluntary groups

There are many voluntary groups concerned in protecting children. The old established ones include Barnado's, the Children's Society, National Children's Homes, and Family Service Units. They have a general concern with child welfare, and much of their work consists of small local projects in various parts of the country.

There are other voluntary organisations, established more recently, that act as advocates, pressure groups or legal advisors to one of the many groups that might be involved in child protection cases, and these would include the Family Rights Group and Parents Against Injustice, the Children's Legal Centre, the National Association of Young People in Care, and Childline.

The National Society for the Prevention of Cruelty to Children (NSPCC) has been in existence now for well over a century, playing a key role in protecting children. It has a national network of field social work staff. There has been a recent shift in their role, away from investigative work and towards preventative and therapeutic work. They have developed expertise in training and research. They produce some excellent publications and in 1997 started a major national campaign to draw the general public's attention to child abuse.

Activity
Select a recent highly publicised child abuse case, and read all the press cuttings. Identify all the agencies and professionals involved.

The role of the child-care practitioner

All child-care practitioners working in any type of setting need to adopt a professional approach to child protection. Working with young children on a day-to-day basis you are one of the most likely people to recognise that abuse is occurring. This can be a very distressing and painful area of your work, and you need to be well prepared, both psychologically and cognitively, to be able to deal with it with sensitively, keeping the best interests of the child in the forefront of your practice. It is very important that you understand and value the role of all the agencies and the other professional people in this area of work, so that you co-operate and work with them as a team to ensure the protection of the children in your care.

GOOD PRACTICE

When working in a multi-disciplinary team, adopt a professional approach.
1 Have a clear understanding of your own role and of the function of your establishment, whilst recognising and understanding the roles of other professionals involved.
2 Communicate effectively with the team.
3 Take advantage of any joint training schemes or discussion groups, as this would help overcome ignorance and prejudice.
4 Respect differences in values and understand that there is a common goal.

One of the many notices that circulates within teams of people states the following message.
'The six most important words in our language are "I admit I made a mistake."
The five most important words are "You did a good job."
The four most important words are "What is your opinion?"
The three most important words are "Let's work together."
The two most important words are "Thank you."
The single most important word is "We." '

Male child-care practitioners

All child-care training incorporates equality of opportunity into the curriculum and most colleges welcome male candidates on to their child-care courses for the positive male caring role they show to the children, for challenging the stereotype of an all-female profession and, it is hoped, for raising the occupational status of child care. Recent research from the Thomas Coram Research Unit has addressed the issue of the recruitment of men on to child-care courses. Child protection is an issue often raised when looking at men working with children and this has been highlighted by the Hunt report into the Jason Dabbs case, where a male child-care student in Newcastle was found to have abused over sixty children while on placement. Males working with very young children may fall under suspicion of abuse more easily than female practitioners.

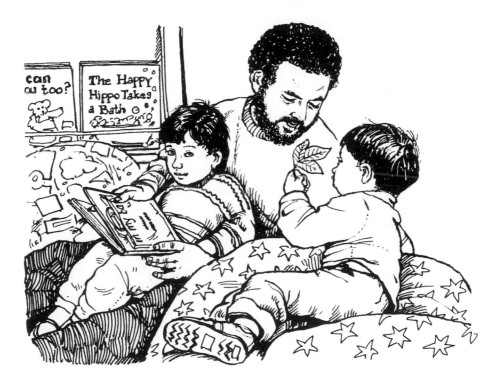

Male child-workers challenge the stereotype of an all-female profession

Colleges should be more rigorous about the procedures and policies agreed with placement supervisors and more alert to the possibilities of students of either gender abusing children. Colleges should be proactive rather than reactive, and prepare both students and placements for the possibilities of abuse.

KEY TERMS

You need to know what these words and phrases mean. Go back through the chapter and make sure that you understand:

designated teacher
duty to investigate
guardian *ad litem*
male child-care workers

multi-disciplinary team
power to protect
statutory duty
voluntary groups

Resources

Cameron, C., 'Men wanted' in *Nursery World*: 15.5.97

Department of Health, *Working Together Under the Children Act*, 1991

Dodd, C., 'Should men work with children?' in *Nursery World*: 21.9.95

Levy, A., (Ed), *Focus on Child Abuse, Medical, Legal and Social Work Perspectives*, Hawkesmere Ltd, 1989

Moss, P., 'Conference report: a man's place in the nursery' in *Nursery World*: 27.6.97

Murphy, M., *Working Together in Child Protection*, Arena, 1995

Whitney, B., *Child Protection for Teachers and Schools*, Kogan Page, 1996

7 FACTORS CONTRIBUTING TO CHILD ABUSE AND NEGLECT

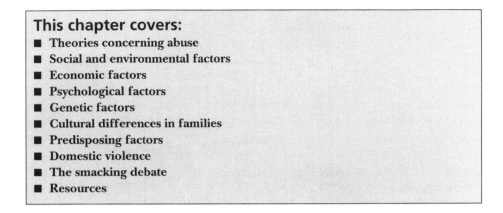

This chapter covers:
- Theories concerning abuse
- Social and environmental factors
- Economic factors
- Psychological factors
- Genetic factors
- Cultural differences in families
- Predisposing factors
- Domestic violence
- The smacking debate
- Resources

There are many factors that contribute to abusing and neglecting children. One thing is very clear: abuse is not restricted to any particular class, culture, race, religion or gender. In spite of this, many people have tried to build a picture of a perpetrator and the factors which may lead to abuse and neglect. What has become obvious is that no one professional or agency can work alone and that we must work together as a community to identify and prevent child abuse and neglect.

Theories concerning abuse

Many theories have been put forward over the last fifty years or so as to why some children are abused or neglected. One popular theory is based on the work that John Bowlby carried out on attachment. Bonding is the term (first used by Spitz in 1945 and made popular by John Bowlby in 1958) for the emotional attachment a mother feels for her new-born baby and the dependency of the baby on the mother. More recently, the term has been used to include both parents.

It has been suggested that separating the mother from the baby immediately following the birth, for whatever reason, may interfere with the bonding process and, therefore, mothers are encouraged to touch and talk with their babies as soon as possible, even if the baby is in an incubator. Fathers are encouraged to be present at ante-natal preparation classes and at the birth, as this is thought to strengthen family relationships. In some cases of neglect and rejection, on looking back it is often apparent that, along with other negative factors, bonding did not satisfactorily take place. It would be foolish to imply from this that if the bonding does not happen immediately the child is at risk, for, in the vast majority of cases, the bonding takes place later on, as it does with adopted children.

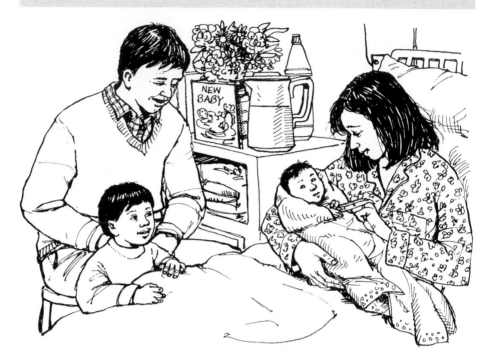

Many theories place great emphasis on bonding

Bowlby suggested that people who may have suffered from poor bonding and maternal deprivation as children are likely to have difficulty in acting as parents in later life, holding unrealistic expectations of their children and often resorting to ill treatment. In many of the enquiries into the death of young children, the perpetrator was found to have been abused as a child. However, one should not necessarily conclude that all abused children go on to abuse as adults.

Another school of thought would suggest that inequalities within society such as poverty, poor housing, unemployment, lack of education, and lack of family and community support may lead to alienation, depression and poor parenting, but it has been shown that all types of abuse take place in all socio-economic groups.

Feminists might argue that a patriarchal society leads to abuse. Children are seen as possessions and are at the disposal of the male members of the household. However, it is clear that both sexes abuse both boys and girls.

Sometimes one child in the family may be abused and treated as a scapegoat. There may appear to be no good reason for this, but it could be that the child is a step-child, or has a disability or learning difficulties, or is, perhaps, a painful reminder of a past or present partner.

Current thought is that the reasons for child abuse must be looked at as a combination of social, psychological, economic and environmental factors. Abuse is found across a wider range of people than these individual theories would have us believe.

Social and environmental factors

The homes and lives of children in the UK have changed dramatically in the last twenty years. There are many possible reasons for this:
- increase in divorce and the number of households headed by one parent
- increase in mobility, so that young families do not always have the support of an extended family, and especially of grandparents
- increase in the number of reconstituted families, and in the number of different relationships that the custodial parent might have
- increase in stress, due to unemployment, uncertainty in employment or longer hours in the workplace
- increase in the number of children living in relative poverty
- increase in drug and alcohol abuse
- increase in violence on television, film and video
- increase in reporting of violence in the media, leading to fear of children gaining independence outside the home and over-shielding them from danger
- increase in house-husbands/partners
- increase in the involvement of the father in some aspects of child rearing
- increase in the number of smaller families so few children grow up with opportunities to learn about baby and child care through direct observation.

In some ways, the home has become a more claustrophobic place. Children do not have the freedom to play outside, even in their own gardens, and spend more time in front of computers, televisions and videos.

Activity
Watch your favourite 'soap' over the course of two weeks.
1 What issues are depicted that might be seen as indicators of the changes in our society?
2 Look at a young child depicted in one of the 'soaps'. If you were a child-care practitioner looking after that child, what elements in that family might you be concerned about?

Economic factors

Being poor does not, in itself, make parents more abusive and most parents living in very deprived circumstances do not abuse or neglect their children, but the added stress that poverty brings may be a contributing factor. Lack of money means poor housing and fewer outings for the children, and the media shows a relatively affluent life style as the norm.

People who have a reasonable income are able to buy in domestic help and child-care support systems. Those with more money and easier access to higher education have a better understanding of how the system works, and are able to take advantage of this. They are more aware of state entitlements, and are more articulate in demanding help.

Lack of money can lead to an impoverished diet, inadequate clothing and poor health. Coping with frequent illness in children or chronic illness in parents or children, leads to even more stress. Parents need to be in good health to cope with the demands of bringing up children.

Social workers, who can alleviate some of the stress of poverty by recommending day-care places and other services, are often unaware of problems in families who appear to be coping and do not seek help.

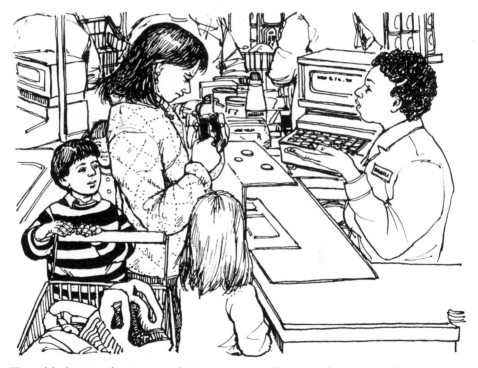

The added stress that poverty brings may contribute to abuse or neglect

Those people who are well-educated and have good job prospects are less likely to settle down in a relationship at a young age, and may defer having children until they are financially stable. They are unlikely to experience unwanted pregnancies as they may well have a better understanding of contraception.

It is important to avoid stereotyping abusers as young, unmarried, poor, or drug or alcohol abusers as these groups are much more open to scrutiny by social services and other professional workers than other groups.

To think about
Consider and discuss the following two statements.
1 Government policies which allow children to grow up in poverty and deprived circumstances should be seen as a type of child abuse.
2 High unemployment levels in any society increase the incidents of child abuse.

CASE STUDY

Robert is 4½, small for his age and pale. He is disruptive and has a very short concentration span. His sister, Emma, is just 3 and is also small and pale with blonde wispy hair. They are both attending your nursery class and arrive in unsuitable dirty clothing, Emma, in particular, smelling of urine. Their mother is often drunk, even early in the mornings. She frequently complains of poverty and begs for money, stating she cannot feed the children, and on one occasion threatened to cut her wrists in front of the children if some money was not forthcoming.

1 What immediate help might you give the children?
2 What short-term help might be available for this family?
3 What long-term help might be found?

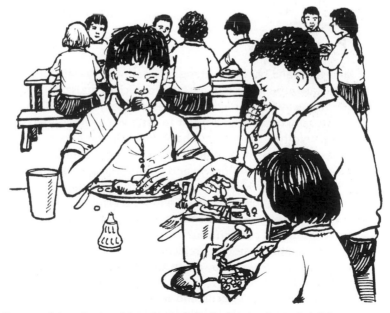

Providing nutritional school lunches can help the neglected child

Psychological factors

It could be the psychological make-up of one parent that leads to abuse or neglect. Psychological factors might include:

- being brought up in a hostile family environment, so that it is difficult to learn how to make loving relationships
- having excessive dependency needs, so that a relationship will be kept going at any price, including domestic violence
- having a large number of children, in the hope that one will finally be the perfect child, while being unable to care for the needs of even one properly
- having unrealistic expectations of children, not understanding their pattern of development and their limitations
- being excessively rigid and obsessive about routines, tidiness and the home environment, while having little understanding of the chaos children can cause
- being unable to cope with stress
- being mentally ill
- being dependent on tranquillisers, drugs or alcohol
- experiencing closeness only after an episode of violence – this may relate to the adult's own childhood.

To think about
Does a parent exist who has not at one time or another been cruel to or neglected his or her child?

CASE STUDY

James is $3\frac{1}{2}$ and has been attending your nursery class for six months. The family are affluent, living in a large detached house. James's father is frequently away from home and James is usually collected from the class by an 'au pair'. It has been difficult to establish a relationship with Felicity, James's mother. She seems to have very little time for or patience with James, often describing him in a disparaging manner. James is becoming quieter and more withdrawn and on one occasion describes being locked in a cupboard for what seemed to him to be all day. When his mother arrives to collect him that day she looks tearful and upset, and smells of drink. James runs and clings to his mother, who pushes him away.

1 What factors concern you?
2 How might his mother's rejection affect James's emotional development, and in what way might this threaten his later achievement at school?
3 What are James's needs, and what are the family's needs?
4 What might you do to help James and his family?

Genetic factors

On 14 February 1997, Professor Emlen of Cornell University, in a controversial paper, suggested that the decline of the nuclear family, and the growth of single parent and reconstituted families was linked to an increase in delinquency, truancy, child abuse and neglect. He suggests that although no gene for caring has yet been discovered many species take more care of their immediate children because they have more of the same genes than strangers and unrelated children. Studies of birds and mammals (including humans) have shown that parents and grandparents tend to help their children effectively, protecting the genes that they have passed on to them. A number of contentious theories have been proposed which attempt to explain why relationships between parents and their biological children may be 'different' from those between carers and non-related children.

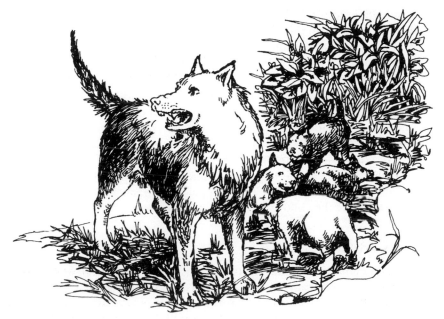

Why do animal mothers care for their own young more than unrelated young?

Activity
Identify any other theories you may have heard which try to explain poor parenting.

Cultural differences in families

Families differ in their attitudes to child rearing practices. What might be thought of as encouraging independence in one family might be looked at as dangerous practice in another. The areas of difference are mainly:

- discipline and control
- independence, both physical and emotional
- providing a safe environment
- diet, which includes attitudes to a 'fussy eater', providing an appropriate diet and using food as a reward or for comfort
- attitude to education
- provision of active play in or out of the home
- mutilation of the body such as ear piercing, circumcision and tribal marks
- attitude to nudity
- employment of children
- demonstrating affection
- sleeping patterns, sharing beds or sharing rooms
- tolerance of crying babies and children
- attitude to noise made by children
- ambitions for their children
- relationship with their children
- treating boys differently from girls
- religion
- moral guidelines.

The variations between families in the ways the children are brought up are many and it is important that you recognise the differences and not leap to conclusions, thinking, for example, that certain religious or ethnic groups always behave in a particular fashion. These variations between and within families lead to the richness of today's diverse society.

Although one has to be non-judgemental and open-minded and avoid stereotyping, if you feel that abuse is taking place in a family you must challenge this, as the interests of the child are paramount.

To think about
It is thought by some that sexual abuse is found more often in families who are not open about sexual matters. Do you agree with this?

Activity
Some families allow their children more freedom and autonomy than others. List the advantages and disadvantages of allowing young children to make their own decisions.

Predisposing factors

It is very difficult to predict the circumstances in which abuse takes place, nevertheless many researchers have suggested that there may be some predisposing factors in individuals. These may relate to the adult's personality and background, problems in the adult's life and environment, and factors relating to the child (Beaver et al, Stanley Thornes, 1994).

A combination of some of the following facts are usually found in abusers:

- young parents reacting to situations in an immature manner, often lacking self-control and coping skills – there may be poor parent with child interaction
- parents who were abused themselves, who have a poor self-image, low self-esteem and poor parenting skills – they may well have unrealistic expectations of the child's abilities and developmental stages
- family stress where, for example, there is a crying baby in the house, unemployment or chronic illness
- inability to control anger
- social isolation, with little backup from the family or the community
- substance abuse
- reconstituted family
- previous abuse, particularly if the original abuse was sadistic
- separation after birth may be associated with abuse
- learning difficulty and/or poor education
- inability to enjoy life and experience pleasure
- unsatisfactory social and personal relationships
- fear of 'sparing the rod and spoiling the child'
- social problems: poverty, poor housing and unemployment
- the gender of the child
- overwhelming personal problems, such as ill health and bereavement.

Activity
Which of the above factors might be found in all social classes?

To think about
We need to put more resources into research into the prevention of child abuse. Do you agree?

The NSPCC has attributed vulnerability factors in child abuse and neglect to the child or to the parents.

THE VULNERABLE CHILD

Born too soon
- born before parents emotionally ready for the child
- statistically more likely to have been born prematurely – weight lower and vulnerable to ill health; more difficult to handle and causes more anxiety

Born sick or handicapped
- abnormal pregnancy, abnormal labour or delivery, neonatal separation, other separation in first six months, illness in first year of child and/or mother

- difficult to feed – growth failure related to physical abuse, unsuccessful feeding may precipitate assault

Born different
- parents' perception of difference is the one that is important

Born unwanted
- unwanted pregnancy
- unwanted gender
- actual child, disappointing replacement for loss of previous child or someone precious

THE VULNERABLE PARENTS

Unhappy childhood
- low self-esteem, more isolated, more life stresses, physical violence or fragile relationships
- may expect criticism and rejection or resent authority

Early parenthood
- youth and immaturity leading to unrealistic expectations of the child
- lack of practical knowledge
- child expected to meet parents' needs

Psychological problems
- no consistent pattern
- parents showing psychiatric symptoms of stress at time of abuse
- attempted suicide of mother
- bereaved parents
- loss during pregnancy, may have relationship problems with new born

The table on page 115 shows some conditions and developmental stages of small children that may trigger abuse.

Domestic violence

Domestic violence features in over a quarter of reported violent crimes, but many incidents will remain unreported. The majority of violence is inflicted by the male partner on the female partner and in a study carried out by the National Children's Home Action for Children in 1994, 83 per cent of the men were father to one or more children in the home. Domestic violence is the second most common type of violent crime reported to the police and is found in all classes and cultures.

Violent men often threaten to harm their children as a way of controlling their partners. In 90 per cent of incidents children were in the same room or in one next door when violence took place.

WHAT PLACES CHILDREN 'AT RISK' OF CHILD ABUSE?

The 'seven deadly sins' – conditions and developmental stages that may trigger physical abuse of small children

Condition/trigger	Description	Age of most danger	Common abuse injuries associated	Advice for stopping/preventing abuse
Colic	All babies show some 'fussy' crying that is inconsolable. About one baby in ten will cry like this frequently and persistently in ways parents find impossible to stop, and for long periods.	1–3 months and then stops	Internal bruising in head, grab-mark bruises, broken arms, legs and ribs	1 Check for any medical causes and then reassure parents this is normal and will stop at about three months or before. 2 Help them to learn soothing techniques and give permission for them meeting *their* needs for sleep and time away from the baby.
Habitual night crying	Some babies develop a habit of waking in the night even after they no longer need a feed. They get to enjoy the extra attention /or find it difficult to sleep without parental care.	4 months – 2 to 3 years	Injuries as above	1 Stop naps during the day, move cot to baby's own room and make bedtime calm. 2 Make 'check-up' visits short, boring and at long intervals. 3 Give more attention and stimulation during the day.
Clinginess and separation anxiety	At about six months a baby comes to depend upon his/her main caregiver(s) for security and will show clinginess and anxiety when separated. Some parents do not understand and see this as the child being spoiled.	6 months – 3 to 4 years	Spanking and slapping injuries. Emotional cruelty e.g. locking up	1 Explain that this stage is normal and necessary for healthy development. 2 Help parents to make separation easier for child – by rehearsal, making it gradual etc. 3 Make sure child is always left with somebody they know, like and trust.
Curiosity and exploration	Children as they develop mentally and physically increasingly explore their surroundings as they become more mobile. Unchecked they can expose themselves to danger. Some parents expect them to follow adult rules and punish them for damaging property or making messes.	1–3 years old	Too little control – burns, poisonings etc. Too much control – bruised from spanking and rough grabbing	1 Explain that exploration and curiosity are natural and necessary parts of growing up. 2 Safety-proof the home and draw up rules for protection, develop firm but non-abusive strategies for managing behaviour. 3 Provide an environment that allows plenty of opportunities to explore.
Disobedience and negativism	As children begin to develop a sense of independence, they often test this out by being disobedient and negative. Parents may feel very threatened by this disobedience.	1½–3 years	Slaps and punches to body and head. Cruel emotional punishment may include locking up, taunting, etc.	1 Explain the phase is normal however irritating. 2 Go for minimal rules and non-confrontation. 3 Offer child choices where possible but don't bargain where there is no choice.
Fussy eating	Because growth slows down, a child's appetite falls off somewhere between eighteen months and two years. Refusing to eat may become a child's way of self-assertion.	1½–3 years	Slap and pinch marks on face and injuries to mouth from force feeding. Children may choke or suffocate.	1 Explain that it is usual to eat less at this age and reassure that the child is fit and well. 2 Cut down on snacks and drinking too much milk. 3 Take the 'heat' out of mealtimes.
Wetting and soiling	Children gain control over their bladders and bowels only gradually. Parents may expect to toilet train too soon or see wetting and soiling as deliberate disobedience.	1–3 years	Bruises, burns and scalds around bottom and genital areas.	1 Advise parents to wait until child is ready for toilet training. 2 Don't attempt to train child at times of stress. 3 Be sympathetic about 'accidents'. They are very seldom deliberate.

The 1994 report found that short-term effects of this violence on the children included:

- problems at school
- difficulty in making friends
- emotional difficulties, such as withdrawal, aggression, displaying fear and anxiety.

The long-term effects included:

- lack of self-confidence
- poor social skills
- violent behaviour
- depression
- difficulties in forming relationships
- disrupted education, resulting in failure to reach their potential.

Many mothers were frightened about revealing the extent of the violence to anyone, through guilt and from fear that the children would be taken away. One of the recommendations following this research was that all children living in violent situations must be considered 'children in need' under the Children Act. A social worker should assess their needs in order to offer support, counselling and therapy.

Children who live within the shadow of domestic violence are often attacked and abused by the offender and without the example of a loving caregiver may go on to become abusers themselves.

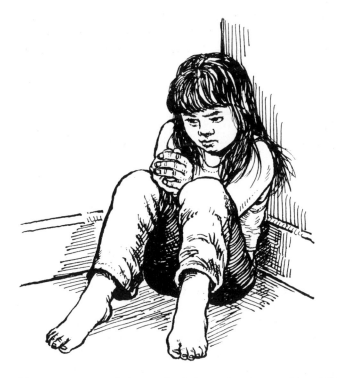

Ninety per cent of domestic violence is witnessed by children

The smacking debate

During the last decade there has been much debate on whether to smack children or not. The UK is one of the last countries in Europe to allow parents and carers to smack children indiscriminately, short of inflicting serious injury. Hitting anyone else is a criminal assault.

The protagonists line up on different sides. One side includes the End Physical Punishment of Children (EPOCH) which was set up in 1989. It now has sixty organisations linked to its campaign, including the NSPCC, the National Children's Bureau, and Save the Children. All the major children's charities support EPOCH's 'commitment to non-violence in parenting, child care and education'. The Gulbenkian Foundation Report on Children and Violence in 1995 proposed a national charter of non-violence. The Chairman of the commission was quoted as saying:

> *Hitting people is wrong. Hitting children teaches them that violence is the most effective means of getting your own way. We must develop a culture which disapproves of all forms of violence. All the lessons of my working life point to the fact that violence breeds misery. It does not resolve it.*
>
> *Sir William Utting*

The opposing arguments are often presented by parents, who contend that 'smacking never did me any harm'. They may quote the Bible, saying that if you spare the rod, you spoil the child. Many parents feel it would be an infringement of their parental rights to legislate against the way they choose to discipline their children. Anne Davis, a childminder and spokesperson of 'Families for Discipline', won the right to smack, in a legal battle against Sutton Borough Council in 1995 after they threatened to de-register her for refusing to sign a form undertaking not to use any physical discipline on children in her care.

As a professional person, looking after other people's children, in the opinion of the authors it is never correct to administer physical punishment, whether the parents request it or not. A light slap is one end of the continuum of beating a child and causing injury, and there would never be any reason why a child-care practitioner should hit a child.

In your working career, you will often come across parents who choose to use physical chastisement to discipline their children. You must use your judgement as to when you feel it is necessary to intervene.

Many parents, who see themselves as 'anti-smackers', may have, on occasion, lost control and administered a slap. They know it is not the way they want to behave, and often feel guilty about it afterwards. Young people, who are not parents, might find this hard to understand.

'Discipline' is frequently thought to be of a physical type. Parents sometimes need help in understanding that there are alternative modes of control.

Activity

How might you manage the following situations?

1 An older child deliberately provoking his younger brother into losing his temper and throwing food onto the floor.
2 A 3-year-old refusing to go to bed, although obviously very tired.
3 A 3-year-old wanting a bath rather than a shower, and refusing to co-operate.
4 A 6-year-old taunting and teasing children from a different culture.
5 A child demanding sweets in a busy supermarket.
6 Three children quarrelling and fighting in a car.

When you start to work with children who are abused and with their families, it will become apparent that there are many factors contributing to the abuse or neglect. All cases are complex and some are never fully understood.

KEY TERMS

You need to know what these words and phrases mean. Go back through the chapter and make sure that you understand:

attachment
bonding
cultural differences
domestic violence
economic factors
EPOCH
genetic factors
inequalities

maternal deprivation
patriarchal society
predisposing factors
psychological factors
smacking
social and environmental factors
vulnerability factors

6 Do not question the child, as other agencies will have to interview the child and information may become distorted.

7 Reassure the child that you will protect and support them.

8 Respect the child's privacy and rules of confidentiality but never promise to keep secrets that you are duty bound to report. Let the child know that you are having to talk to someone else.

9 Follow the procedures for reporting and investigating the abuse, as set down in your workplace.

10 Make sure that the language you use is appropriate to the child's level of understanding, and that you do not put ideas into the child's head.

11 Make an immediate timed, dated and signed record of the conversation.

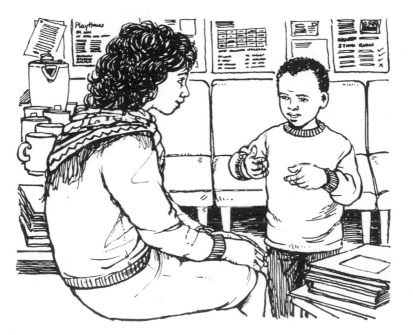

Listen to the child, but do not press for information

Record-keeping

If at all possible find a quiet place and endeavour to write an accurate record of the conversation, being scrupulous in leaving out your own feelings, and in being objective. Make a note of the date, time and the place where the conversation was held. Make a note of any dates and times mentioned, and the key phrases used by the child. If the child uses euphemisms, such as 'willy', write down those, rather than interpreting the words yourself. These notes and records must be made within twenty-four hours if they are to be legally admissible. When giving this record to your line manager, make sure you make a copy for yourself, and keep it in a safe and secure place. The procedures of the establishment will now be followed. You should try to do some careful observations of the child's behaviour and record any conversations which might take place, during the time of the investigation.

Communicating with colleagues

COMMUNICATING WITH THE TEAM IN THE WORK SETTING

Because of the constraints of confidentiality, your discussions about any concerns you have about a particular child will be limited strictly to those who need to know. For example, you will have informed your line manager as soon as the child has disclosed to you. If you are working in a school, the headteacher and the designated teacher will also be in consultation. In a nursery or pre-school you will inform the person with overall responsibility, and the same is true in a day-care centre.

Care should be taken that conversations are held privately, and that documentation is stored safely under lock and key. It goes without saying that no one will indulge in gossip about the child or the family.

You will need to keep all lines of communication open as the case is referred to the social services, and the procedures are put into operation. It is hoped that this communication will allow you to be fully informed of events and developments as they take place, so that you can do your best when planning work with the child and the family.

To think about
Policies on how to deal with disclosure may vary in different establishments. Discuss these differences with your group.

COMMUNICATION WITH OTHER AGENCIES

Since the inquiry into the death of Maria Colwell, the failure of communication between the agencies involved in child protection work has been seen in some cases to contribute to serious injury or even death. Subsequent inquiries have reinforced the critical importance of good multi-disciplinary communication in preventing and recognising abuse and neglect.

Research has indicated that good multi-disciplinary communication is facilitated by:
- all professionals feeling valued for their contribution
- good inter-personal skills, involving active listening and clear articulation without the use of jargon
- valuing and respecting the work of others
- good inter-disciplinary training

- understanding each others' roles
- recognising and challenging stereotyping and racism
- dealing calmly with conflict
- never attempting to take over another agency's work.

Since the Children Act, 1989, a greater emphasis than previously has been placed on the need to communicate well with parents.

Confidentiality

There may be conflict among some professionals when a child discloses and asks them not to take the information further. This issue has been addressed by Childline who offer children complete confidentiality unless they are in a life threatening situation. On occasion, very serious incidences of sexual abuse have led to the police being informed. Children know that they are in control of the situation, and that it is up to them whether they wish the matter taken any further. As a child-care practitioner you are unlikely to have children in your care who are old enough to request confidentiality.

Expressing yourself at child protection conferences

If you are invited to attend a conference because you have information and observations concerning a child, you will probably find yourself quite anxious. Your line manager or designated teacher may be invited to attend with you and you will have the opportunity to discuss your contribution beforehand. The best way to ease your worries is to be well prepared and organised. You will receive general information and an agenda prior to the meeting. Make yourself familiar with everybody's role and make sure you understand the procedures.

Remember:
- accept that you will be nervous beforehand and brush up on the relaxation techniques that work for you
- be positive and confident in your role
- monitor your vocal expression, thinking about volume, pitch and speed, and take your time
- articulate your words more clearly than usual, as you are speaking to a larger group
- prepare any written statements, observations or general notes prior to the conference so that you can use them usefully in response to questions
- make copies of anything you may wish to distribute prior to the conference, confirming with your line manager that you are not breaching confidentiality
- if you should suddenly go blank, pause, take a breath, refer to your notes and carry on – this happens to most people at some time
- most people present will feel anxious and this may be expressed in different

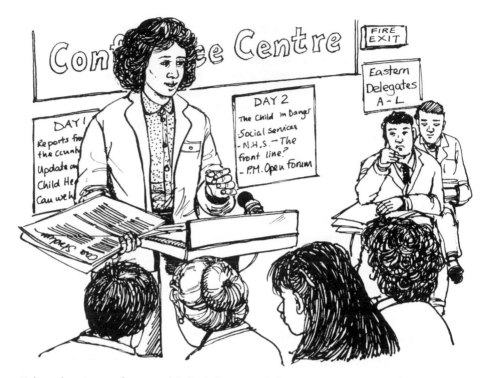

Take advantage of any multi-disciplinary training

ways – an experienced chairperson will understand this and attempt to keep the meeting focused
- the parents may be present
- some explicit terms may be used that you might find embarrassing to express or to hear – prepare yourself for this; when you are reporting the terminology of the child it is important that you repeat the exact words said to you
- concentrate on the task – you are there to communicate an important message from the child.

If you have not been invited to attend, or it is impossible for some reason for you to do so, send in a report.

Throughout your course, taking part in group discussions and contributing to seminars and debates will prepare you well for this type of activity in employment.

Giving evidence in court

In the unlikely event that you may be asked to go to court as a witness, you should be well prepared for your task beforehand. It is worthwhile having knowledge of court procedures in advance. There may well be a delay between the incident and the court hearing. It is essential that your notes and records are as full as possible. You are allowed to use informal notes that you have made for your own benefit in court.

With the best will in the world, court proceedings often involve a great deal of waiting around. You may be given a specific time to attend rather than being expected to be there for the whole of the proceedings, but many delays can occur, or the proceedings can be cut short. Occasionally, the hearing is rearranged or re-scheduled. It is advisable to take something to occupy yourself, such as a book or a journal.

If you have to appear in court, this will probably be at the instigation of the local authority, and you will have to make a statement to their solicitor. You may have to describe events that you have witnessed, or your observations of the child's behaviour. The solicitor should advise you, and your line manager should be available to support you through the process. This is particularly important after the appearance, when you will want to discuss and reflect on the experience.

Care proceedings concerning child protection cases are informal and not open to the general public. All those involved sit at the same level. No one is on trial. Everyone has the same mission: to identify the best interests of the child.

Activity

In your group, take it in turns to read out a general observation you have made during your time in your present placement. You do not have to choose an observation on a child about whom you are concerned. Expect questions by the group, and try to prepare your answers in advance. This will enable you to practice standing up before a number of people, and being questioned on your report.

GOOD PRACTICE

When attending court, be well prepared and organised.

1 Acquire as much information as you can before the event.
2 Make sure your record keeping is always meticulous and up to date, and remember to take all your records and notes with you.
3 Look neat and tidy, and be punctual.
4 Listen carefully to any questions. Reflect for a moment before you respond as clearly as possible.
5 Be objective. Stick to the facts, unless an opinion is sought.
6 Be truthful, and do not elaborate or waffle.
7 If you do not understand, ask for the question to be repeated. If you still do not understand, say so.
8 Concentrate on the question in hand. Try not to anticipate the next question.

Feelings

Whenever you read in the media about a small child being abused or neglected, your feelings are aroused. How much more so if the abuse should happen to a child in your care?

Initially, you will be shocked and horrified, and may view the evidence of abuse with some disbelief. As you begin to accept the situation you may experience waves of anger, revulsion and disgust towards the perpetrator. Then the professional side of you will take over and you will realise that your job is to help the child and the family come to terms with what has happened, and that your observations and reports will be objective and valuable at child protection conferences and in court if necessary. You will probably feel apprehensive and nervous if you are asked to give evidence, particularly if you were the one the child disclosed to, or who picked up the evidence of physical abuse. When first working in a multi-disciplinary setting you may feel some reluctance to contribute to arguments produced by highly qualified knowledgeable professionals. It is important that you remember that you are the professional in daily contact with the child and are there to make sure the voice of the child is heard.

At first, the people to whom you reported the abuse might not have been convinced, and you may have experienced feelings of frustration at not being able to put the case across sufficiently well to ensure that the child was protected.

It has been said that 10 per cent of the population have suffered some form of abuse or neglect, and if you were one of these the discovery of abuse would re-invoke the feelings you had in the past, and might make it more difficult for you to accept that abuse is occurring and take action but, as a professional, you know you have to put your own feelings on one side and act in the interests of the child.

Discovery may arouse strong feelings of guilt, firstly because you had not recognised the abuse earlier, and secondly because you were slow to accept what was happening. You might feel that you could have prevented the abuse in some way. This would not be true, and none of it is your fault. You are not the perpetrator.

If the abuser is someone you know and have built a relationship with, it often destroys your faith in humanity for a short while. If the perpetrator is one of the parents, you have to get over your feelings of anger and betrayal and your reluctance to communicate with him or her. You will need to remain on professional terms, so as to help the child. Remember that most parents do love their children and want the best for them. Focus on the needs of parents rather than the injuries of the child. You should not be surprised by repeated rejection from the parents, who lack self-esteem and trust, and who are experiencing fear, guilt and remorse. Be careful not to over-identify with the parents so that your objectivity becomes affected.

Some staff may find it difficult to remain working in an establishment following a court case, and the numbers of staff resigning may rise.

Christina Maslach, a leading American researcher in the field of stress, has identified several key factors in contributing to the anxiety felt by practitioners working with abused children.

- Issues around child abuse are always complex, with families suffering from multiple problems within society, and in their personal relationships. It is hard to lay down rules which would apply across the board, as each case is unique.
- Statistics show that many child-care practitioners have themselves been the victims of abuse, and contact with abused children and their families may well trigger painful feelings and suppressed memories from childhood.
- In trying to help these families you are exposed to people who are angry, despairing, suspicious, resentful and frustrated. They may well vent these feelings on you.
- Lack of resources, inadequate training and work overload make many long-term cases difficult to deal with.
- The rules of confidentiality that may have to be set aside in the interests of the child, can result in a conflict of interest.

Dealing with stress

Managing a child in your care who requires protection may result in a great deal of stress. It is in the best interest of the child that you are aware of the stress, and know how to deal with it. All courses that train child-care practitioners will have covered stress management.

Activity
List under the following three headings the physical, the psychological and the behavioural indicators of stress. Check your answers with Appendix 3 at the end of the book.

Unlike most incidents which bring a great deal of stress, resigning from your post would not be the answer here. You have a professional duty to the child and the child must come first. There are various coping strategies which will help you to reduce the level of stress.
- Discuss the issues with your line manager or designated teacher openly and honestly, not attempting to disguise your own feelings. Their experience may help you to recognise and learn to live with the strength of your feelings.
- A clear action plan agreed with your line manager will help you to feel more positive and reduce the uncertainties inherent in the situation.
- You may be fortunate enough to have access to personal counselling, where you can express your feelings and opinions. This is particularly important if you have been a victim of abuse or neglect in the past.
- Talking through the situation with a close trusted friend to whom you do not, of course, disclose the identity of the family or the child, can be very helpful and supportive.

- Taking advantage of training, either in general stress management techniques or child protection training that addresses this area of concern can be of advantage.
- Remember you are there for all the children and try not to allow the needs of one child to dominate so that the others do not get a fair share of your time. Make your day as normal as possible.
- Try to leave the stress behind you in the workplace. Try hard to relax on your days off.
- Exercise regularly to relieve tension and discover a relaxation technique that works for you.

During your training you will have acquired many communication skills, and will have profited in using them in all areas of the work: with children, with parents and with colleagues. When protecting children, you need to be a particularly skilled listener, be able to express yourself clearly, in speech and in writing, to parents, colleagues and to other professionals.

KEY TERMS

You need to know what these words and phrases mean. Go back through the chapter and make sure that you understand:

communication	interviews
confidentiality	leading questions
coping strategies	professional duty
disclosure	record keeping
effective listening	social listening
feelings	stress
giving evidence in court	voice of the child

Resources

Alsop, P. and McCaffrey, T., *How to Cope with Childhood Stress*, NSPCC, 1996
Bannister, A., Barret, K. and Shearer, E., *Listening to Children*, NSPCC
Barnado's (8 minute video): 'You're Going to be a Witness', £55 from Bridgewater Project. Telephone 01642 300774
Burnard, P., *Communicate! A Communication Skills Guide for Health Care Workers*, Edward Arnold, 1992
Elliott, M., *Keeping Safe: a Practical Guide to Talking to Children*, Coronet, 1994
Haynes, M., *Effective Meeting Skills*, Kogan Page, 1988
Jay, A. and Jay, R., *Effective Presentation*, Pitman Publishing, 1996
Kelcher, M., *Better Communication Skills for Work*, BBC Books, 1992
Leigh, A. and Maynard, M., *Perfect Communications*, Arrow Books, 1994

Makin, P. and Lindley, P., *Positive Stress Management*, Kogan Page, 1992

National Early Years Network, *Keeping and Writing Records*, 1994 (booklet)

Petrie, P., *Communication with Children and Adults*, Edward Arnold, 1989

Taylor, M., 'The art of communication' in *Nursery World*: 7.12.95

9 WORKING WITH ABUSED CHILDREN

> **This chapter covers:**
> ■ Behavioural characteristics
> ■ Your role in the prevention of abuse
> ■ Working with abused children
> ■ Children with disabilities
> ■ Supporting children in the criminal court
> ■ Play therapy
> ■ Child advocacy centres
> ■ Resources

The vast majority of children that you will be working with in your career as a child-care practitioner will come from stable happy homes where you will work in partnership with the parents to meet the needs of the children and promote their all round development. There are some children who are not so fortunate and if you are working with these children you will play a key role in identifying abuse, observing the children and helping them to recover from the effects of abuse and neglect.

Behavioural characteristics

The effects of abuse on young children in the short-term have been described in chapter 5, 'Following recognition of abuse'. In their study of 50 abused children, Martin and Beezley (1977) describe some characteristic behaviour:

■ impaired capacity to enjoy life: abused children often appear sad, preoccupied and listless
■ symptoms of stress, for example, bed-wetting, tantrums, bizarre behaviour and eating problems
■ low self-esteem – children who have been abused often think they must be worthless to deserve such treatment
■ learning difficulties, such as lack of concentration
■ withdrawal – many abused children withdraw from relationships with other children and become isolated and depressed
■ opposition or defiance – a generally negative, uncooperative attitude
■ hypervigilance, described as frozen awareness or a watchful expression
■ compulsivity – abused children sometimes feel or think they must carry out certain activities or rituals repeatedly
■ pseudo-mature behaviour – a false appearance of independence or being excessively 'good' all the time or offering indiscriminate affection to any adult who takes an interest.

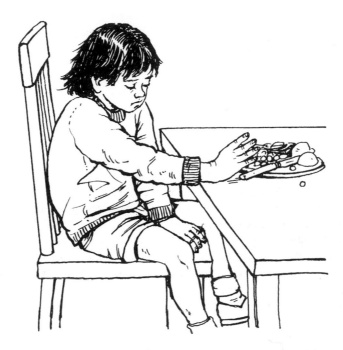

Abused children may exhibit stress symptoms, such as eating problems

These behaviour patterns can also be looked upon as indicators of abuse. Children may react by becoming aggressive or withdrawn.

Your role in the prevention of abuse

Because of the dire consequences to children who are abused, the whole community: parents, professionals, neighbours, and politicians, share the responsibility of prevention and attempting to secure the safety of young children. Your role, as a child-care practitioner, is to:
- be alert and watchful
- be knowledgeable, understanding the predisposing factors and indicators of abuse
- teach children to protect themselves by giving them information, awareness and coping skills
- help parents to understand normal child development, and not to have unrealistic expectations of their young children
- help parents to manage children's challenging behaviour in a positive manner
- recognise situations when parents may be under stress and offer help when possible.
- be a good role model, presenting a calm professional manner when you yourself feel upset or stressed.

As child-care practitioners, in whatever setting you are working, your planning of activities should include areas where you can encourage children to protect themselves. Teach children:

- the difference between comfortable and uncomfortable touches
- that safety rules apply to all adults, not just strangers
- that secrets they feel uncomfortable about should be discussed with a trusted adult; any hugs or kisses given by an adult and told to be kept secret should always be disclosed
- to feel good about themselves, and know that they are loved and valued
- to trust, recognise and accept their own feelings
- that their bodies belong to them, and nobody has the right to touch or hurt them
- that they can say 'no' to requests that make them feel uncomfortable, even from a close relative or family friend
- that they can rely on you to believe and protect them if they confide in you
- that they are not to blame if adults hurt them
- that people should not be categorised as 'good' or 'bad' – it is more important to teach children about the danger signs than to watch out for 'bad people'
- that rules of good behaviour can be broken if they feel they are in danger, and it is perfectly all right to fight, kick, bite, punch, shout and scream if they feel threatened

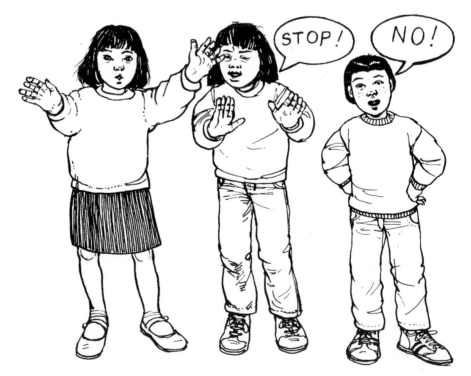

Help children to learn that they can say 'no'

- that they can tell you of any frightening incident, assuring them that you will listen and believe what they say and will never be angry with them
- that they can help to deal with bullies by being more assertive; if they cannot cope with the bully, they must tell an adult
- that they must not to talk to strangers, even when the stranger appears kind and says he or she knows the parents; always tell a supportive adult and never go off with someone they do not know.

There are outside agencies who are willing to come and talk to the children in your care about protecting themselves. The one which is most well-known is Kidscape which was founded in 1984 to enable children to learn about personal safety and teach them strategies to keep themselves safe. There are also books and teaching aids, some of which are listed at the back of this book and some at the end of the chapter. The NSPCC, among others, produces a wealth of helpful material such as leaflets, posters and brochures.

Activity
Design an activity for 6- to 7-year-olds, to assist in the prevention of abuse.

Working with abused children

Abuse and neglect have a severe effect on the all-round development of the children involved. An abused child will have strong emotional feelings, which will get in the way of learning and discovering the environment.

A child who has experienced positive and consistent parenting will have had the opportunity to explore his or her environment, to make trusting relationships with peers and other adults, and have enough self confidence to persist in the pursuit of knowledge, in spite of set-backs. Language will be encouraged and stimulated, and will be a valuable tool in finding out about the world.

Not all children are abused within the family, and a supportive and loving family background helps the child come to terms with what may have happened.

To think about
What is the role of the child-care practitioner in supporting parents who wish to keep their children safe?

A small minority of children who have been abused may be referred to a play therapist. Because play therapists are in short supply, significantly more children will benefit from the skilled attentions of a child-care practitioner. The best way of helping will be to understand and encourage the child to express his or her feelings, either in speech or in activities that allow emotional expression, and to empower the child to have control over his or her environment.

Children who have been abused may experience many different emotions, many of them overwhelming. These feelings will depend on their age and on their level of experience.

- Fear:
  of the abuser
  of making trouble
  of losing a significant adult in their lives
  of being taken into care
  of being different from other children.
- Isolation:
  because 'something is wrong with me'
  because they feel on their own
  because it is difficult to talk about the experience.
- Anger:
  at the perpetrator
  at the other adults who failed to protect them
  at themselves, feeling that they are somehow to blame.
- Depression expressed by:
  lack of self-esteem
  lack of confidence
  under achievement
  withdrawal from friends and adults.
- Guilt:
  for not stopping the abuse
  for allowing the abuse in the first place
  for disclosing the abuse
  for not disclosing the abuse.
- Sadness:
  at losing part of their childhood
  at losing part of themselves
  at losing trust.
- Shame:
  at consenting to the abuse.
- Confusion:
  because they may still love the abuser
  because their feelings are in constant turmoil
  because they find it difficult to establish new trusting relationships.

Most activities in the pre-school, in particular, are designed to give children confidence and a sense of achievement, give them power and control over their environment, and develop their expressive language. Messy play, such as finger painting and clay activities, let children release pent up emotion in a creative way. Playing with dough is calming, as is water and dry sand play, and lets a child spend time reflectively, without any expectations of producing a piece of work. Conversations can take place with a trusted adult when doing sensory activities, and help the child to express his or her emotions verbally. Listening to music and taking part in playing instruments is another outlet for emotion. Making a puppet may encourage a child to say things through the puppet which he or she might otherwise hold back. Using stories on a one-to-one basis can also be helpful. Domestic play in the home corner, where a child feels private and invisible to adults, creates an enabling environment which may encourage the child to act out his or her feelings. It is important to provide dolls in the home corner for the child to interact with. For some children, physical activity and outside play may help with suppressed emotions.

It cannot be emphasised enough how important it is to continue to monitor the child with observations, record keeping and assessment. Your skills in these areas are highly valued:

- observe the child at all times
- listen attentively to what the child is saying
- hear what the child does not say
- consider and evaluate the child's behaviour
- plan positively to help the child, tailoring the daily activities to the current needs of the child
- give the child a great deal of attention and encouragement.

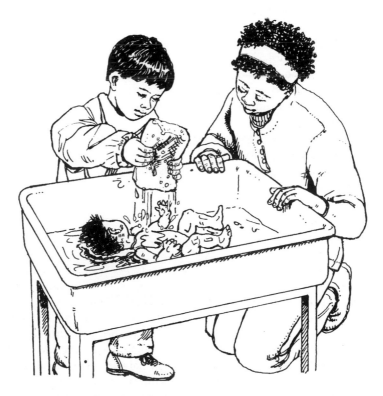

Provide dolls for the child to interact with

Maintain professional standards in your work with abused children.

1 Keep up to date with current practice and procedures.
2 Have a good understanding and knowledge of child development, and understand how this can affected by abuse and neglect.
3 Display empathy and understanding.
4 Encourage trusting relationships. If the child wishes, respond to the child's need to be held and cuddled.
5 Be professional, and do not feel threatened or distressed by the child's expression of emotions.
6 Establish and maintain a professional relationship with the parents/carers.
7 Give extra time to the child whenever you can on a one-to-one basis.
8 Provide activities every day to allow emotional expression and encourage communication.
9 Have realistic expectations of the child's progress and development. Each small step should be seen as an achievement.
10 Create situations where the child can succeed.
11 Encourage the child to be responsible for others. Taking care of the class/nursery pet helps a child to feel empowered and of value.
12 Accept challenging behaviour. Show disapproval of the action rather than the child.
13 Set limits for the child, as allowing any aberrant behaviour will make a child feel insecure.
14 Value the views and opinions of the child and involve him or her in decision making and in becoming more assertive.
15 Show the child that you care for him or her, but resist the temptation to over protect.
16 Always touch the child gently, and be aware of any movement that the child might see as threatening.
17 Maintain professional standards of observation, evaluation and planning.
18 Maintain liaison with the multi-disciplinary team.

Activity

Design and make an appropriate resource, such as a book, a game, a comfort toy or a puppet, to help a child come to terms with and recover from abuse.

Children with disabilities

In 1996 the National Children's Bureau reported that there were 360,000 children under 16 with a disability. Of these 5,500 lived in residential care, whilst 16,000 attended residential schools. It is very hard to obtain accurate figures for disabled children who suffer abuse in this country, as very often a disability is not mentioned in the reports of abuse. Studies in America appear to indicate that disabled children are more at risk, as the overall incidence of abuse among disabled children is 1.7 times higher than in the general child population, and these children were found to be twice as likely to experience emotional neglect and physical abuse.

Children with disabilities, particularly those with speech or learning difficulties, are more vulnerable to abuse. This is because:

- they have communication difficulties and are therefore less able to report the abuse
- their parents/carers might be dependent on respite or long-term care, and are not always fully aware of what might be happening to their children
- there may be some problem in recognising indicators of abuse, as these might be attributed to the disability
- people might be less inclined to believe that a disabled child was abused
- the behaviour of the child may be very challenging, and lead to a lack of control on the part of the parent/carer
- a child who does not seem to respond to love and affection might deter the parents/carers from persevering in meeting the child's needs
- children are more vulnerable if they are in institutional care
- the children's requirements for intimate care make them vulnerable.

P. Newport (1991), *Linking Child Abuse with Disability*, published by Barnardo's, expanded the definition of abuse for disabled children to include:

- lack of stimulation
- over protection
- confinement to room or cot
- lack of supervision
- incorrectly given medication
- insensitive, intrusive or disrespectful applications of medical photography and medical rehabilitation
- parents' failure to acknowledge or understand the disability
- parents' unrealistic expectations

Other definitions include:

- force-feeding
- neglect of medical care
- deprivation of aids
- physical restraints
- teasing and bullying within the community.

If you are working with children with a disability, either in the mainstream school, the special school, day care or the home, the same good practice as outlined previously is relevant, but obviously requiring more skill and knowledge of the impairment. You will also have to carry out more intimate care for the child such as:

- toileting
- bathing, and skin and hair care
- feeding
- dressing and undressing.

Until you have established a good and trusting relationship with the child, it is advisable to allow a preferred adult to perform such tasks. This may not always be possible, especially if you are working as a nanny. Whatever the situation, make sure that you treat the child with respect and sensitivity working towards the empowerment and independence of the child.

Activity
What disabilities would make a child most vulnerable to abuse? Why?

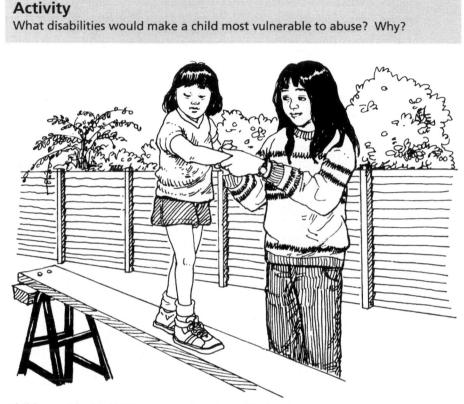

Children with disabilities are more vulnerable to abuse

Supporting children in the criminal court

Although this country has come some way to alleviating the distress of a court appearance, by videoing evidence at pre-trial hearings, a child may still have to attend court to give evidence if the defendant pleads not guilty. The stress often leads to the prosecution being abandoned, or the case not coming to trial in the first place. One proposed suggestion is the use of adult supporters, usually a social worker or a person drawn from voluntary organisations, with a similar brief to that of the guardian *ad litem* in civil cases to advise and support the child, safeguarding his or her interests.

An adult supporter may:

■ assume overall responsibility for the welfare of the child witness, before, during and immediately after the trial

- explain the process to the child, appropriate to age, understanding and mode of communication – this does not mean rehearsing the evidence or discussing its content
- ensure appropriate facilities are made available to the child before and during the trial
- liaise with parents/carers, local authorities, police, and the crown prosecution service
- arrange a prior visit to the court, enabling the child to practice speaking in court with the means of a live television link.

You, as a child-care practitioner, will make yourself as familiar as possible with the court proceedings, so as to be able to answer questions and reassure the child as much as possible.

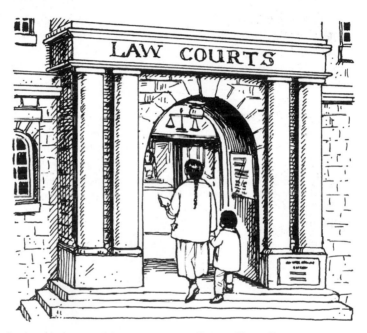

A child who has to cope with court proceedings will need support

Play therapy

In the UK the focus of attention on child protection is often prevention, recognition, investigation and possible legal intervention. Less emphasis is placed on therapeutic strategies to help the child recover. Very few children find themselves referred to a skilled play therapist and, with the younger children, a great deal of the work can be done by the child-care practitioner. A number of books are being written about the role of the play therapist, and should be used as a reference by child-care practitioners who work with children who have been abused.

Ann Cattanach looks at the value of play linked with a number of child development theorists and has some excellent ideas for specialist activities.

> *The play therapy process for the abused child is an exploration through play which helps the child make sense of her experiences in a way which is appropriate to her developmental level. The form and content of the exploration is determined by the child and there are many and varied ways for the child to use play.*
>
> *Ann Cattanach*

She defines three stages in the play therapy process:

- *The establishment of a relationship between the child and the therapist, so that trust is engendered and the transitional space between the therapist and child is a safe place for exploration. The therapist can become aware of the specific problems presented by the child at this stage.*
- *The child and therapist explore through toys, objects, and dramatic play, in a more focused way, to help integrate and make sense of some of the horror of the past. There is much repetitive play at this stage.*
- *The child is helped to develop self-esteem and an identity not so bound up in the abusive relationships of the past.*

> *Ann Cattanach*

Play specialists have access to a large collection of puppets and dolls, some of which may be anatomically correct. The children may be familiar with the latter as they may have been used when collecting evidence during an investigation, and videos have sometimes been made of children using these dolls to demonstrate the abuse they have suffered.

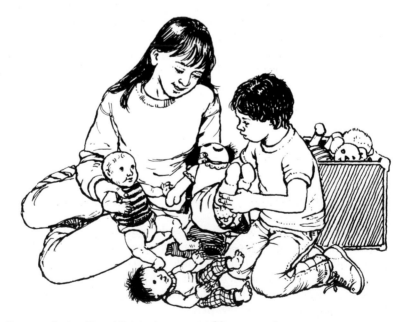

Play therapy helps the child make sense of her experiences

Child advocacy centres

In the USA, Child Advocacy Centres have been opened, mainly in the cities, so that all the agencies who deal with child sexual abuse are under one roof: police, lawyers, social workers, medical examiners and therapists. At a conference held in the UK, in Herefordshire in May 1997, it was stated that two types of therapy were offered: crisis therapy and long-term therapy. The child receiving therapy was thought to remain more 'intact', and more able to deal with the situation. The case of Declan Curren was sited. He was a teenager who hanged himself. He had asked for counselling after being sexually abused and, as it was not immediately available, had not been able to come to terms with the abuse. The disadvantages against such centres were:
- the child was interviewed in a strange place, not in his or her own home
- strangers would do the examination, not the child's own GP
- rural areas would be difficult to cover adequately.

The American results showed that:
- probably more abusers were caught
- the children's lives were made better, as the child's self-image was strengthened immediately
- information was shared in a speedier and more accurate manner.

To think about
Child advocacy centres may be opening in the UK. What advantages or disadvantages would there be for children in your area?

As a child-care practitioner, you will have developed a warm, trusting relationship, and the toys and objects you will be working with will be familiar to the child. The room in which you work will be a safe haven and will help the child to relax and enjoy the play you feel will be most helpful. The great advantage of a play therapist or of a child advocacy centre is that long sessions of time working with the child on a one-to-one basis are available, whereas you will have other children to care for and duties to fulfil.

KEY TERMS

You need to know what these words and phrases mean. Go back through the chapter and make sure that you understand:

activities
characteristic behaviour
child advocacy centres
children with disabilities
comfortable and uncomfortable
   touches
emotions
empowerment
independence

Kidscape
observations, record keeping and
   assessment
play therapy
prevention of abuse
secrets
supporting children
therapeutic strategies

Resources

Books to use with children

Hessell, J. *What's Wrong with Bottoms?*, Hutchinsons Children's Books, 1987

Peake, A. and Khadj, R., *My Book, My Body*, The Children's Society, 1989

Pre-school Press, *It's OK to Say 'NO'*, Colouring and Activity books, Pre-school Press, USA, 1985

Books for reference

Alsop, P. and McCaffry, T., *How to Cope with Childhood Stress*, NSPCC, 1996

Axline, V., *Play Therapy*, Churchill Livingstone,1989

Brock, E., *Child Abuse and the Schools' Response: a Workshop for Professionals Involved with Young People*, NSPCC

Butler, I. and Roberts, G., *Social Work with Children and Families: Getting into Practice*, Jessica Kingsley, 1997

Cattanach, A., *Play Therapy with Abused Children*, Jessica Kingsley, 1993; *Play Therapy: Where the Sky Meets the Underworld*, Jessica Kingsley, 1994; *Children's Stories in Play Therapy*, Jessica Kingsley, 1997

Childline, *Going to Court: Child Witnesses in Their Own Words*, 1996

Cloke, C. and Naish, J., *Key Issues in Child Protection*, NSPCC and Longman, 1992

Dixon, D., *Teaching Young Children to Care: 37 Activities for Developing Self-esteem*, Twenty-third Publications, USA, 1990

Doyle, C., *Working with Abused Children*, Macmillan, 1990; *Helping Strategies for Child Sexual Abuse*, National Children's Bureau, 1996

Elliott, M., *Feeling Happy, Feeling Safe*, Hodder and Stoughton, 1991; *Female Sexual Abuse: the Ultimate Taboo*, Pitman Publishing, 1996

Findlay, C. and Salter, A., *Protecting Children and Young People*, Skills for Caring Series, Churchill Livingstone, 1992

Freeman, L., *Loving Touches*, Parenting Press Inc. Seattle, USA, 1986

Gil, E., *The Healing Power of Play: Working with Abused Children*, Guilford Press, USA, 1991

Glaser, D., *Child Sexual Abuse*, Macmillan, 1993

Hobart, C. and Frankel, J., *A Practical Guide to Activities for Young Children*, Stanley Thornes (Publishers) Ltd, 1995

Jessel, C., *If You Meet a Stranger*, Walker Books, 1990

National Early Years, *Young Children Under Stress*, 1992 (booklet)

Sanders, P., *Feeling Safe*, Lets Talk About Series, Gloucester Press, 1987

West, J., *Child Centred Play Therapy*, 2nd Ed, Arnold, 1996

Westcott, H. and Cross, M., *This Far and No Further: Towards Ending the Abuse of Disabled Children*, Venture Press for the British Association of Social Workers,1996

Whitney, B., *Child Protection for Teachers and Schools*, Kogan Page, 1996

10 WORKING WITH PARENTS

It is part of the professional practice of child-care practitioners to work closely with parents, communicating effectively and regularly, respecting their greater knowledge of the child, and involving them in all decision making. The Children Act, 1989, emphasises the need for partnership with parents and, where possible, enhancing and not undermining the parents' role.

Helping parents to understand abuse

Most children are abused by adults known to them. This could be the father or the mother, a step-parent, a grandparent, an older sibling, or any member of the extended family. It could also be someone in whom the parents have placed their trust, such as a neighbour or a baby-sitter, a sports coach or regrettably even the child-care practitioner. Because this is the case, it is always more difficult for the child to acknowledge that the abuser is someone they know and probably love. If a child is severely neglected, this abuse would obviously be the responsibility of the parents, as they are the ones expected to meet the needs of the child.

Some people might think that children are over protected today because of the parents' fear of strangers abducting and sexually abusing their children. Statistically, 'stranger abuse' is a minuscule part of the whole area of abuse but nevertheless, parents should be taught that to keep their children safe they need to:
- know where their children are at all times
- be sensitive to changes in their children's behaviour and look out for any indicators of abuse
- listen carefully to their children and discuss any underlying worries
- teach them to say no
- teach them to trust their feelings, if they feel uncomfortable with anyone
- check out carefully any adult they entrust their child to, such as childminders and baby-sitters
- be alert to any person over attentive to the child, or giving inappropriate gifts.

Child-care practitioners will support parents in their relationships with their children by encouraging them to:

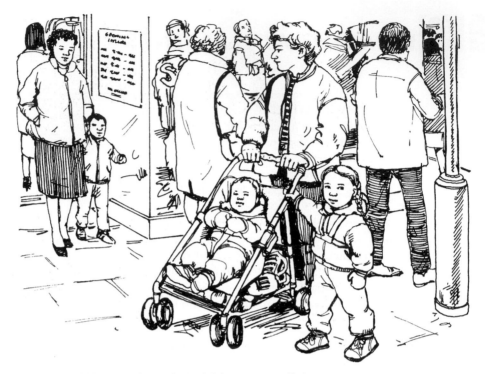

Parents should know where their children are at all times

- meet the children's basic needs and ensure their physical care, safety, and healthy development
- show and express love to their children
- communicate regularly and listen sensitively
- foster moral, social and spiritual development, helping the children to establish a clear set of values
- establish clear consistent daily routines
- set boundaries to their children's behaviour and be consistent
- empathise with the children
- praise and encourage the children, and attempt to ignore challenging behaviour
- answer their children's questions, and encourage their curiosity and need to obtain knowledge
- respect and value the children, and apologise when in the wrong
- have fun and enjoy their children
- have time for themselves, and do not exclude their own needs
- have some understanding of child development and age-appropriate behaviour
- have regular contact and communication with the staff team.

It is especially important that you work in partnership with black and ethnic minority families, who often experience discrimination and may well have different

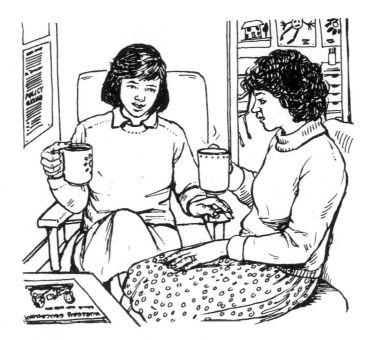

Offer support and encouragement to parents

child-rearing practices than those with which you are familiar. You need to have a sound knowledge of the culture of all the families with whom you are working. P. Mares, A. Henley and C. Baxter suggested in 1985 that if professionals are to work in partnership with black and ethnic minority families to prevent child abuse in our multiracial and multicultural society, they will need to think seriously about the following questions.

- How far are you seen by the family as a friend and confident?
- How far are you seen as representing the law, or a form of social control?
- Does the family understand your role and that of other professionals?
- By what value and criteria is the family being assessed and judged?
- Do you carry with you any stereotyped and unhelpful notions?
- Is the system quicker to remove black and ethnic minority children from their families and what is your role in supporting families through this?

The rights and responsibilities of parents

The Children Act, 1989, states that parents have a number of key rights and at the same time a number of important responsibilities. A new concept of parental responsibility is defined in the Act as 'all the rights, duties, powers, responsibilities and authority which, by law, a parent has in relation to a child and his property'. Parents' rights under the Act include:

- the right to have a say in any decision-making about their child
- the right to have their views heard in court cases involving their child.

These rights and responsibilities apply to parents, whatever their situation, whether they are married or divorced. Although an unmarried father does not automatically have parental responsibility, he can acquire it if the child's mother agrees or if a court says so. If a court decides a child needs to go into care to be protected, the local authority gains parental responsibility, but must share this with the parents and negotiate how it will be exercised.

The Act emphasises the importance of partnership in looking after children. Partnerships should be formed between social services departments and parents. Social services departments must listen to the views of parents for whom they are providing a service and give them a say in how their child is cared for. Parents with a child in need can best serve his or her interests by working with social services departments to get the help and support they need.

Parents have the right to:
- be informed about actions being taken that concern their child
- put their case in court
- be involved in the decision-making about their child when he or she is being looked after by the local authority
- have the court resolve disputes over contact with the child
- be told of any applications to court (unless the situation is so serious that the local authority must act immediately).

It can be seen that the Children Act has spelt out for parents their rights and responsibilities, and you will need to be conversant with the Act when working with parents.

The child-care practitioner as role model

As a child-care practitioner, you are a carer and an educator. These are the same roles that parents fulfil, and by your example, children and parents can learn from you how to care and form relationships with other people. As a professional person, you will naturally show respect and a positive regard for the welfare of the children in your care at all times.

There are certain situations that parents find stressful. The NSPCC has named seven stress behaviour situations as:

- the child who will not stop crying
- defiance and disobedience
- children squabbling
- temper tantrums
- unfavourable comparisons with other parents by the child
- refusing to go to bed
- moodiness and argumentativeness.

Activity

How many more stressful situations can you think of? What strategies might you teach parents to understand and cope with this behaviour?

By the way you react to such situations with patience and empathy, you are teaching a very valuable lesson to the young people in your care. Many of the skills you display are the skills that children will need when they are parents. Your appropriate response to challenging behaviour will have an impact on the child, and will be seen to be fair by all the children in the group. Your meticulous attention to equal opportunities will ensure that all children reach their potential and are not trapped in stereotypical roles. The way you listen carefully to what both children and parents have to impart, will show how much you respect and value their views and opinions. You will be able to advise families if they are going through stressful

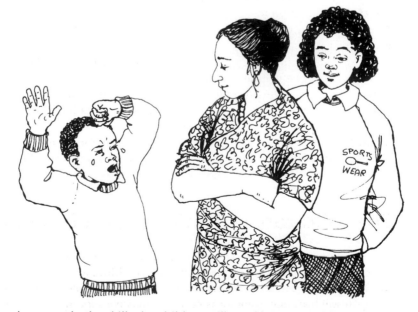

Show by example the skills the children will need later on in life

times, pointing out helplines like Parentline, and finding out about local information for parents and carers. Most boroughs have leaflets especially written for parents, often in many different languages. You will reject violent responses to situations, and show children how to respond in an assertive fashion rather than resorting to aggression. Observing and assessing children's individual needs will show you which children might need some individual attention from time to time, while you always have time for all the children in your care. You will at all times display a commitment to equal opportunities and anti-discriminatory practices. It is natural to respond more to some children than to others, but you will, of course, not allow yourself to show any favouritism.

By attempting to adopt this pattern of behaviour at all times, you will be showing by your example the skills the children will need later on in life when they become parents themselves.

Worrying behaviour that might cause concern

All families behave differently, and some of the following factors might occur, from time to time, in families where there is no question of abuse. A number of these signs exhibited over a period of time should cause concern:

- frequent smacking and shouting at babies and children, often for behaviour that is developmentally normal, such as a toddler wetting his or her pants
- expecting the child to be the parent, giving love and comfort to the adult
- parental indifference to the whereabouts and safety of their children
- barking orders at a child, without displaying patience or clear explanations of what is expected
- never giving praise or encouragement
- unreal expectations of appropriate behaviour
- discouraging the child's natural curiosity, and not providing enough stimulation
- seeing the normal behaviour and actions of a child as a deliberate act to upset and annoy the parents
- frequent rows and disagreements between the parents and other family members, perhaps leading to violence.

To think about
Should parenting skills be taught as part of the National Curriculum?

Working with parents who have abused

One of the most useful things you can do is to show parents how to cope with the needs of children and their sometimes challenging behaviour. All children are lively, and challenging adults is part of their development. It is unrealistic to expect small children to be quiet and well behaved day in and day out. Physical abuse is occasionally caused by parents/carers under stress not being able to cope with what is really quite normal behaviour, particularly if they are depressed and isolated. You, if working as a nanny, may well have experienced some of these feelings yourself, but being a professional trained person you will have the resources to cope with them. Encourage the parents to respond by:

- taking a deep breath and counting to ten
- remembering they are mature, and do not need to react like a child
- understanding and re-directing their anger, perhaps by punching a pillow
- remembering that young children can often be diverted by offering another activity
- going into another room for a short time, away from the child, collecting their thoughts and giving themselves time and space to evaluate the situation
- contacting someone on the telephone to express their feelings
- using local resources, such as drop-in centres and parent centres
- going outside to scream and shout and let their feelings out, out of sight and hearing of the child
- trying to keep a sense of proportion.

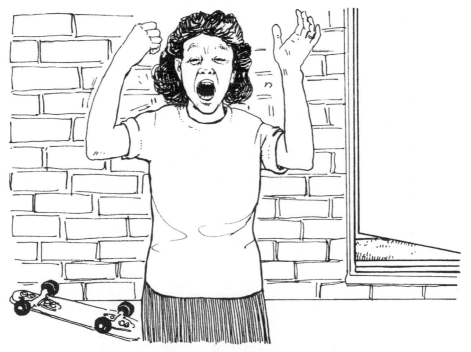

Sometimes it helps to go outside to let off steam

To think about

What do you think should happen if a 7-year-old has been physically abused and neglected, yet does not wish to leave his family and live with foster carers?

If the person suspected of committing abuse is one of the child's parents, the other people in the family will need your support and advice, as they will be confused and upset about what has happened. They may need someone to talk to who will listen in a non-judgemental way, or they may need information and help. They will be very important to the child's eventual recovery, and you will need to be as sensitive and supportive to them as possible.

You may be working with children where abuse and neglect has been diagnosed whilst they are attending your establishment, or social services may request a placement for a child as part of a child protection plan. In some areas of the country there may be family centres where you may be working with the family together with other members of a multi-disciplinary team, such as psychotherapists and social workers.

CASE STUDY

Andrew

The social worker asked the school if they would admit Andrew into the nursery class, even though his chronological age was 6. Andrew had a much loved older brother, who was developmentally normal. Andrew had been rejected at birth, and his mother refused to feed him.

When he came on the first day, he did not look at all out of place. He was short and thin and you would think he was no more than 3 years old,

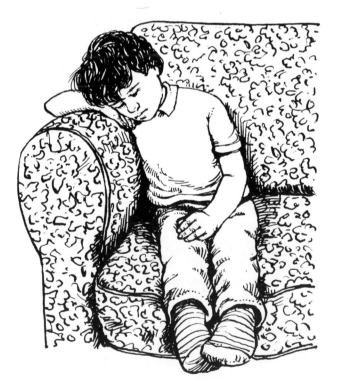

especially when you tried to have a conversation with him. His speech was very delayed, and his comprehension immature. Physically, his muscle tone was poor, and he often fell down for no apparent reason. He spent a lot of the day alone in the book corner, rocking to and fro.

The nursery team gave him three meals a day in the nursery – breakfast, dinner and a cooked tea. This did not help Andrew over the weekends or during the school holidays. Then the mother was asked to attend the mealtimes and, although she was very reluctant at first, she was eventually persuaded to help prepare the meals, and to sit with Andrew while he ate. This seemed to break the cycle of neglect and she came to accept Andrew as part of the family.

1   Why might some mothers neglect their children?
2   In settling Andrew into the nursery, how would you try to involve Andrew's mother into the process?
3   What particular observations might be helpful?
4   How might you prepare Andrew and his mother for entry into the infant school?

Whatever the type of abuse, if you find yourself in the position of working with parents who have abused, you will attempt to:

- acknowledge your feelings and seek opportunities to express them appropriately with colleagues and line managers
- always remember that you need to work with the parents for the good of the child, and therefore need to establish a working relationship
- avoid colluding with the parents through fear of aggression
- deal with the isolation the situation might demand
- talk and liaise with the other agencies concerned with the case
- be aware of the child protection plan for this family
- record conversations and decisions taken with the family, using plain jargon-free language
- request supervision of your work by a competent line manager
- acknowledge and relieve the stress of the whole family.

Remind yourself that when you are working with parents you are helping the child and playing a part in breaking the cycle of abuse. Try to assume a non-judgemental attitude and refrain from questioning the parents about the abuse, or from challenging information they may give you, as this is the task of other agencies. If the parents are coming to your establishment as part of a child protection plan, take time to introduce them to the unit and to the routines, giving them as much information as possible about the care of the child. Listen to what they are saying and express appropriate concern and kindness whilst remaining objective and empathetic. You will need to foster the parents self-respect and improve their self-image. It is hard for parents to understand where they have gone wrong and they have to cope with the close scrutiny of their parenting practice by many different people, finding it often difficult to have a clear idea of what they are meant to achieve. Although the task is challenging for the child-care practitioner, you will not be working in isolation and it is very worthwhile.

Encourage good parenting skills.

1 Present yourself as a good role model, in all areas of child care. Use a non-threatening approach at all times.
2 Build a trusting relationship with the parents, working with their strengths rather than weaknesses.
3 Use praise and encouragement as positive reinforcement, when the parent shows appropriate behaviour.
4 Work with the parents in planning the child's future care and development.
5 Listen to the parents, and try to establish what particular areas of care they find most trying.
6 Explain to the parents which behaviour of the child is quite normal for the stage of development.
7 Give help and information in dealing with any behaviour the parent finds difficult.
8 Discuss the importance of a consistent response, and suggest appropriate and alternative ways of socialising the child.
9 Promote equality of opportunity.

It is understood that working with abused children is very demanding and stressful. We hope that by writing this book we have clarified the issues and procedures that will help you contribute to the prevention of abuse and neglect, to recognise the signs and indicators of abuse, and to work fruitfully with the children and families who have been affected.

KEY TERMS

You need to know what these words and phrases mean. Go back through the chapter and make sure that you understand:

challenging behaviour
discrimination
equal opportunities
parental responsibility
parenting skills

partnership with parents
role model
'stranger abuse'
stresses of parenthood
worrying behaviour

Resources

Bond, H., 'Living with child abuse' in Nursery World: 11.1.96
Department of Health, *The Children Act and Local Authorities: A Guide for Parents,* 1991; *The Children Act and the Courts: A Guide for Parents,* 1997
HMSO, *The Challenge of Partnership in Child Protection: Practice Guide,* 1995
Hollows, A., *Rebuilding Families after Abuse,* National Children's Bureau, 1995

NSPCC, *Stress: A Guide for Parents*; *Putting Children First: A Guide for Parents of 0–5 Year-olds*

Peake, A. and Fletcher, M., *Strong Mothers*, Russell House Publishing, 1997

Platt, D. and Shemmings, D., *Making Enquiries into Alleged Child Abuse and Neglect: Partnership with Families*, NSPCC, 1995

APPENDIX 1: ACTS OF PARLIAMENT THAT AFFECT CHILDREN

1802 Health and Morals of Apprentices Act: restricted pauper cotton apprentices to 12 hours work a day.

1833 The Factory Act: limited the working hours of children in textile mills and appointed factory inspectors with a right of entry.

1872 Infant Life Protection Act: a reaction to scandals resulting from baby farming, where mothers entrusted their children to women to be looked after for payment. Foster parents had to register with the local authority. An investigatory procedure into the deaths of infants was established. Extended in 1897 to cover children up to the age of 5 years.

1872 Bastardy Laws Amendment Act: supported mother's claim for maintenance from the putative father.

1874 Registration of Births and Deaths: became compulsory.

1889 Prevention of Cruelty to Children Act: following the inauguration of the National Society for the Prevention of Cruelty to Children (NSPCC), this act was passed specifically to protect children. This was essentially a criminal rather than a social welfare approach.

1889 The Poor Law (Children) Act: gave boards of guardians the authority to assume parental rights over abandoned children. This was extended in 1899 to include orphans, children of parents who were disabled or in prison, or unfit to have care of them. In 1904 the responsibility was transferred from the Poor Law guardians to the local authority.

1904 The Prevention of Cruelty to Children: gave the local authorities powers to remove children from their parents, including those who had not actually been convicted of a criminal offence against them, but where it met the needs of the children.

1906 The Education (Provision of Meals) Act: gave the local authority the right to levy a rate to finance school meals for those in need. This followed a report in 1904 when attention was drawn to the poor physique of recruits in the Boer War, and concern was expressed about the lack of good food, good air and good clothes. The Act also required the setting up of Children's Care Committees to look into the circumstances of children needing feeding. Schools for Mothers were established, which later became Infant Welfare Centres.

1906: Huddersfield promoted a private Act for compulsory notification of births within the borough.

1907 Notification of Births Act: gave similar powers to authorities that desired them. This became compulsory in 1915.

1907 Education (Administrative Provisions Act): introduced medical inspection of children in elementary schools. It was the first personal health service to be established by Parliament.

1908 Children Act: concerned with the cases of cruelty and neglect, it attempted to strengthen the powers of the courts for the benefit of the child at risk. It established Juvenile Courts and Borstals to deal with young offenders under the age of 16. Shopkeepers were forbidden to sell alcohol and tobacco to juveniles. Limits were set on the hours children were allowed to work.

1911: maternity benefits were introduced.

1929 Infant Life (Preservation) Act.

1933 Children and Young Persons Act: primarily concerned with treatment of young offenders but also included young people who were the victims of cruelty or other offences committed by adults. Local Education Authorities were now required to investigate such cases and bring them before a court empowered to commit the children to the care of the local authority. The emphasis was on rescue, not prevention.

1938 Infanticide Act: accepted the fact that some women may injure or kill their babies while suffering from severe mental illness associated with childbirth.

1948 Children Act: emphasised the importance of keeping children in the care of their natural family wherever possible. This was a shift from punishing bad parents to acting in the interests of the children. Children's Departments were established, staffed by social workers known as child care officers.

1963 Children and Young Persons Act: raised the age of criminal responsibility from 8 to 10. It enabled the local authorities to use resources, including money, to promote the welfare of the child.

1969 Children and Young Persons Act: increased the priority given to caring for children away from home.

1975 Children Act and the **1980 Child Care Act**: both emphasised care in fostering and adoption.

1989 Children Act: see chapter 2.

APPENDIX 2: PERCENTILE CHARTS

Percentile charts, which were compiled after taking the measurements of thousands of children, are used for recording the weight, height and head circumference of babies and children. There are separate charts for boys and girls.

The thick line labelled 50th in the graph below is the average measurement. The line marked 97th shows weights of boys who are heaviest in their group. As you record a measurement regularly on a chart the line will show you the child's individual progress, and allow you to compare that child with other children.

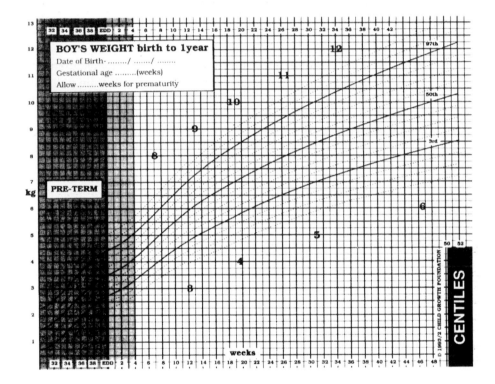

As a rough guide, any child falling below the bottom line on the graph (3rd percentile) should be admitted to hospital for examination. If, when in hospital with no specific treatment, the child gains weight at more than 50 grams a day it is likely that the quality of care has been poor. Most children admitted to hospital for medical reasons tend to lose weight.

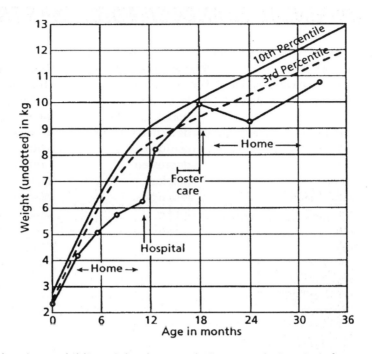

Chart showing a child's weight changes during stays in hospital, foster care and home

APPENDIX 3: INDICATORS OF STRESS

Physical
Aches and pains
Anorexia
Headaches
Dry mouth
Nail biting
Fatigue
Tension
Sexual dysfunction
Fidgeting
Insomnia
Sweating
Palpitations
Back pain
High blood pressure
Nausea
Restlessness
Skin blotches/flushes
Stomach cramps
Lack of co-ordination
Twitching
Shaking
Rapid breathing
Diarrhoea
Constipation
Neck pain
Rigid body
Clenched hands
Gritted teeth
Little eye contact

Psychological
Feeling:
    anxious
    bored
    detached
    confused
    depressed
    helpless
    lethargic
    lonely
    negative
    nervous
    angry
    defensive
    rejected
    isolated
    indecisive
    tearful
Experiencing:
    mood swings
    paranoia
    lack of concentration
    nightmares
    lack of self-control

Behavioural
Over-eating
Under-eating
Increased drinking
Increased smoking
Irritable
Fidgeting
Violent outbursts
Waking early
Unable to organise time
Unsociable behaviour
Aggressive
Cynical
Finding fault
Crying
Inflexible
Isolated
Low sex drive
Nagging
Tantrums
Nervous cough
Nervous laughter

APPENDIX 4: OFFENCES AGAINST CHILDREN

- The murder of a child or young person under 18
- Common assault and battery
- Infanticide
- Child destruction
- Manslaughter of a child or young person under 18
- The abandonment or exposure of a child under two so as to endanger its life or health
- Cruelty (including assault, ill treatment or neglect) to a person under 16
- Allowing a person under 16 to be in a brothel
- Causing or allowing a person under 16 to be used for begging
- Exposing a child under 7 to risk of burning
- Allowing a person under 16 to take part in a dangerous performance
- Rape (or attempted rape) of a girl under 18
- Procurement (or attempted procurement) of a girl under 18 by threats
- Procurement of a girl under 18 by false pretences
- Administering drugs to a girl under 18 to obtain or facilitate intercourse
- Intercourse (or attempted intercourse) with a girl under 13
- Intercourse (or attempted intercourse) with a girl between 13 and 16
- Incest (or attempt to commit incest) by a man against a female, where the victim is under 18
- Incest (or attempt to commit incest) by a woman, where the victim is under 18
- Buggery (or attempt to commit buggery) with a person under 18
- Indecency between men where one, or both, is under 18
- Indecent assault on a girl under 18
- Indecent assault on a male under 18
- Assault with intent to commit buggery
- Abduction of unmarried girl under 16 from parent or guardian
- Causing (or attempting to cause) prostitution of girl under 18
- Procuration (or attempted procuration) of a girl under 18
- Detention of girl in brothel or other premises
- Permitting girl under 16 to use premises for intercourse
- Causing or encouraging prostitution of, intercourse with, or indecent assault on, a girl under 16
- Indecent conduct towards a child under 14
- Aiding, abetting, counselling or procuring the suicide of a person under 18

APPENDIX 5: RESOURCES

Books

Alsop, P. and McCaffrey, T., *How to Cope with Childhood Stress*, NSPCC, 1996

Aries, P., *Centuries of Childhood*, Penguin, 1962

Axline, V., *Play Therapy*, Churchill Livingstone, 1989

Bannister, A., Barret, K. and Shearer, E., *Listening to Children*, NSPCC

Benedict, H., *Stand Up for Yourself*, Hodder Headline, 1996

Bowlby, J., *Child Care and the Growth of Love*, Penguin, 1965

Brock, E., *Child Abuse and the Schools' Response: a Workshop for Professionals Involved with Young People*, NSPCC

Bryant Mole, K., *Bullying*, Wayland, 1994

Burnard, P., *Communicate! A Communication Skills Guide for Health Care Workers*, Edward Arnold, 1992

Butler, I. and Roberts, G., *Social Work with Children and Families: Getting into Practice*, Jessica Kingsley, 1997

Cattanach, A., *Play Therapy with Abused Children*, Jessica Kingsley, 1993; *Play Therapy: Where the Sky Meets the Underworld*, Jessica Kingsley, 1994; *Children's Stories in Play Therapy*, Jessica Kingsley, 1997

Cloke, C. and Naish, J., *Key Issues in Child Protection*, NSPCC and Longman, 1992

Cobley, C., *Child Abuse and the Law*, Cavendish Publishing Ltd, 1995

Corby, B., *Child Abuse: Towards a Knowledge Base*, OUP, 1993

Davies, M., Cloke, C. and Finkelhor, D., *Participation and Empowerment in Child Protection*, Pitman and NSPCC, 1995

de Mause, Lloyd, *The History of Childhood*, Condor Books, Souvenir Press, 1973

Dixon, D., *Teaching Young Children to Care: 37 Activities for Developing Self-esteem*, Twenty-third Publications, USA, 1990

Donnelly, C. (Ed), *What Are Children's Rights?*, Independence, 1996

Doyle, C., *Working with Abused Children*, Macmillan, 1990; *Helping Strategies for Child Sexual Abuse*, National Children's Bureau, 1996

Elliott, M., *Feeling Happy, Feeling Safe*, Hodder and Stoughton, 1991; *Keeping Safe: A Practical Guide to Talking to Children*, Coronet, 1994; *Female Sexual Abuse of Children: the Ultimate Taboo*, Pitman Publishing, 1996

Findlay, C. and Salter, A., *Protecting Children and Young People*, Skills for Caring Series, Churchill Livingstone, 1992

Freeman, L., *Loving Touches*, Parenting Press Inc. Seattle, USA, 1986

Gil, E., *The Healing Power of Play: Working with Abused Children*, Guilford Press, USA, 1991

Glaser, D., *Child Sexual Abuse*, Macmillan, 1993

Haynes, M., *Effective Meeting Skills*, Kogan Page, 1988

Hobart, C. and Frankel, J., *A Practical Guide to Child Observation*, Stanley Thornes (Publishers) Ltd, 1994; *A Practical Guide to Activities for Young Children*, Stanley Thornes (Publishers) Ltd, 1995

Hobbs, C.J. and Wynne, J.M., *Balliere's Clinical Paediatrics: Child Abuse*, Balliere, Tindall, 1993

Hollows, A., *Rebuilding Families After Abuse*, National Children's Bureau, 1995

Horwath, J. and Lawson, B. (Eds), *Trust Betrayed: Munchausen Syndrome by Proxy*, National Children's Bureau, 1995

Jackson, V., *Racism and Child Protection*, Cassell, 1996

Jay, A. and Jay, R., *Effective Presentation*, Pitman Publishing, 1996

Jehu, D., *Beyond Sexual Abuse*, Wiley, 1993

Jessel, C., *If You Meet a Stranger*, Walker Books, 1990

Johnson, P., *Understanding the Problem – Child Abuse*, Crowood Press, 1990

Jones, D.N. et al., *Understanding Child Abuse*, Hodder and Stoughton, 1987

Kelcher, M., *Better Communication Skills for Work*, BBC Books, 1992

Kempe, R.S. and Kempe, C.H., *Child Abuse*, Developing Child Series, Fontana, 1978

Leigh, A. and Maynard, M., *Perfect Communications*, Arrow Books, 1994

Levy, A. (Ed), *Focus on Child Abuse, Medical, Legal and Social Work Perspectives*, Hawkesmere Ltd, 1989

Lyon, C. and de Cruz, P., *Child Abuse*, Jordan, 1993

Makin, P. and Lindley, P., *Positive Stress Management*, Kogan Page, 1992

Mayes, G.M. et al., *Child Sexual Abuse*, Scottish Academic Press Ltd, 1992

Meadow, R., 'ABC of Child Abuse' in *British Medical Journal*, 1989

Moore, J., *The ABC of Child Protection*, Arena, 1992

Murphy, M., *Working Together in Child Protection*, Arena, 1995

Newell, P., *The UN Convention and Children's Rights in the UK*, National Children's Bureau, 1991

O'Hagan, K., *Emotional and Psychological Abuse of Children*, OUP, 1993

Owen, H. and Pritchard, J. (Eds), *Good Practice in Child Protection: a Manual for Professionals*, Jessica Kingsley Publishers, 1993

Parton, N., *The Politics of Child Abuse*, Macmillan, 1985

Peake, A. and Fletcher, M., *Strong Mothers*, Russell House Publishing, 1997

Petrie, P., *Communication with Children and Adults*, Edward Arnold, 1989

Platt, D. and Shemmings, D., *Making Enquiries into Alleged Child Abuse and Neglect: Partnership with Families*, NSPCC, 1995

Pre-school Press, *It's OK to Say NO*, Colouring and Activity books, Pre-school Press, USA, 1985

Pugh, G. and Hollows, A., *Child Protection in Early Childhood Services*, (seminar papers, 1994)

Reder, P., Duncan, S. and Gray, M., *Beyond Blame*, Routledge, 1993

Reid, Dr D.H.S., *Suffer the Little Children (Orkney Child Abuse Scandal)*, Medical Institute for Research in Child Cruelty, 1992

Sanders, A., *It Hurts Me Too*, Childline WAF and NISW, 1995

Sanders, P., *Feeling Safe*, Gloucester Press, 1987

Stainton, Rogers W. and Roche, J., *Children's Welfare and Children's Rights: a Practical Guide to the Law*, Hodder and Stoughton, 1994

Stevenson, O. (Ed), *Child Abuse*, Harvester Wheatsheaf, 1989

Turnabout Distribution Ltd, *Children and Violence*, Turnabout Distribution Ltd, 27 Horsell Road, London N5 1XL

Walker, A., *Possessing the Secret of Joy*, Jonathan Cape, 1992

Waterhouse, L. (Ed), *Child Abuse and Child Abusers*, Jessica Kingsley, 1993

Wattam, C., *Making a Case in Child Protection*, NSPCC,

Westcott, H. and Cross, M., *This Far and No Further: Towards Ending the Abuse of Disabled Children*, Venture Press for the British Association of Social Workers, 1996

Whitney, B., *Child Protection for Teachers and Schools*, Kogan Page, 1996

Wiehe, V.R., *Working with Child Abuse and Neglect*, F.E. Peacock Publishers Inc., ITASCA, Illinois 60143, 1992

West, J., *Child Centred Play Therapy*, 2nd ed, Arnold, 1996

Woodden, K., *Weeping in the Playtime of Others*, McGrath Hill Paperbacks, 1976

Videos

Barnado's, *You're Going to be a Witness*, (8 minutes) £55 from Bridgewater Project. Telephone 01642 300774

NSPCC, *Protecting our Children*, NSPCC with Tower Hamlets Ethnic Minorities Child Protection team, in Sylheti with English subtitles

Helplines

Childline. Telephone: 0800 1111

Child Poverty Action Group. Telephone: 0171 253 3406

Children's Legal Centre. Telephone: 01206 873 820

Contact a Family (for families with disabled children). Telephone: 0171 383 3566

Cry-Sis (counselling advice if you feel your baby cries excessively). London WC1N 3XX. Telephone 0171 404 5011

EPOCH (alternatives to smacking). 77 Holloway Road, N7 8JZ. Telephone 0171 700 0627

Exploring Parenthood (aims to reduce family stress), 4 Ivory Place, 20a Threadgold Street, London W11 4BP. Telephone: 0171 221 6681

Gingerbread (help for single parents), 16–17 Clerkenwell Close, London EC1R 0AA. Telephone: 0171 336 8184

Home-Start UK (practical help for distressed families), 2 Salisbury Road, Leicester LE1 7QR. Telephone: 0116 233 9955 (or see local directory)

Kidscape, 152 Buckingham Palace Road, London SW1W 9TR. Telephone: 0171 730 3300

Meet-a-Mum Association (MAMA) (for mothers suffering from post-natal depression), 14 Willis Road, Croydon CR0 2XX. Telephone: 0181 656 7318

National Children's Bureau, 8 Wakely Street, London EC1V 7QE. Telephone: 0171 843 6000

National Newpin (parenting skills training), Sutherland House, 35 Sutherland Square, London SE17 3EE. Telephone: 0171 703 6326

NSPCC, 42 Curtain Road, London EC2A 3NH. Telephone: 0800 800 500

Parent Network, 44–46 Caversham Road, London NW5 2DS. Telephone: 0171 485 8535

Parentline, Westbury House, 57 Hart Road, Thundersley, Essex SS7 3PD. Telephone: 01268 757077

Relate, Herbert Gray College, Little Church Street, Rugby, CV21 3AP. Telephone: 01788 573241

Save the Children Fund, 17 Grove Lane, London SE5 8RD. Telephone: 0171 703 5400

Stepfamily – National Stepfamily Association (support for all members of reconstituted families). Telephone: 0171 209 2464

The Children's Society, Edward Rudolph House, Margery Street, London WC1X 0JL. Telephone: 0171 837 4299

Research papers, leaflets and booklets

Barnardo's
Getting Positive about Discipline
Splintered Lives (1996)
Why Speak Out Against Smacking?

Childline
Children and Racism
Going to Court. Child Witnesses in Their Own Words (1996)

Children's Legal Centre Briefing
Being a Witness
Child Abduction (information sheet)
Child Sexual Abuse (information sheet)
The Children Act, 1989
Children's Rights after Cleveland
Supporting the Child Witness
The UN Convention on the Rights of the Child

Department of Health, HMSO
The Challenge of Partnership in Child Protection: Practice Guide (1995)
Child Abuse Interventions: a Review of the Research Literature (1993)
Child Abuse: a Study of Inquiry Reports 1980–1989 (1991)
Child Protection: Messages from Research (1995)
The Children Act and the Courts: a Guide for Parents
The Children Act and Local Authorities: a Guide for Parents
Children and Young People on Child Protection Registers (1995)
Children and Young People on Child Protection Registers: year ending 31.3.1996
An Introduction to the Children Act, 1989, (1991)
An Introductory Guide for the NHS: The Children Act, (free, 1992)
Working Together Under the Children Act, 1989 (1991)

Kidscape
Keeping Kids Safe
Protect Children from Paedophiles
Stop Bullying

National Children's Bureau
Child Sexual Abuse, Highlight No. 119
The Children Act,1989, Highlight No. 91
Children and Domestic Violence, Highlight No. 139 (November 1996)
Family Law Act, 1996, Highlight No. 146
An Introduction to Children's Rights, Highlight No. 113
Parental Psychiatric Disorder and Child Maltreatment, Part 1: Context and Historical Overview, Highlight No. 148 (November 1996)

National Early Years Network (Volcuf)
Child Abuse: a Guide for Early Years Workers
Equal Opportunities
Keeping and Writing Records (1994)
Recognising Child Abuse
Young Children Under Stress, (1992)

National Children's Homes Action for Children
Child Sexual Abuse
Messages from Children, (1994)
The Report of the Committee of Inquiry into Children and Young People who Sexually Abuse Other Children (1992)

NSPCC
Child Abuse
Protecting Children from Sexual Abuse in the Community (1997)
Putting Children First: a Guide for Parents of 0–5 Year-olds
Stress: a Guide for Parents

Articles

Barton, C. and Moss, K., 'Who can smack now?' in *Journal of Child Law,* 1994
Bond, H., 'Emotional abuse' in *Nursery World*: 4.8.94; 'Mothers who abduct children' in *Nursery World*: 9.11.95; 'Living with child abuse' in *Nursery World*: 11.1.96
Brazler, C., 'Child labour' in *New Internationalist* magazine, July 1997
Cameron, C., 'Men wanted' in *Nursery World*: 15.5.97
Corke, S., 'A damaging cult' in *Nursery World*: 10.9.92
Dodd, C., 'Should men work with children?' in *Nursery World*: 21.9.95
Elliot, M., 'The ultimate taboo' in *Nursery World*: 2.11.95
Jenkins, P., 'When child abuse is legal' in *Nursery World*: 9.3.95

Moss, P., 'Conference report: a man's place in the nursery' in *Nursery World*: 27.6.97

Mullins, A., 'Relieving the pain' in *Nursery World*: 10.7.97

Neale, B., Bools, C. and Meadow, R., 'Problems in the assessment and management of Munchausen syndrome by proxy abuse' in *Children and Society*, Vol. 5, 1991

Nursery World, 'Not in front of the children' in *Nursery World*: 8.12.92; 'A vicious circle' in *Nursery World*: 2.3.95; 'Tackling child abuse' in *Nursery World*: 16.3.95; 'Why I abuse children' (conference report) in *Nursery World:* 11.5.95; 'Hitting or smacking?' in *Nursery World:* 11.1.96; 'Spanking good news' in *Nursery World Professional Nanny*, November 1996

Stead, J., 'Caught in the net' in *Nursery World*: 3.10.96

Taylor, M., 'The art of communication' in *Nursery World*: 7.12.95

Wallace, W., 'Children who abuse children' in *Nursery World*: 6.7.95; 'Duty of care' in *Nursery World*: 24.10.96; Look who's watching' in *Nursery World*: 25.9.97

Woolfson, R., 'Munchausen syndrome by proxy – the mysterious syndrome' in *Nursery World*: 15.6.89

INDEX

abuse
  by children 60
  in the workplace 86
accidental injury 77
activities 143
anti-discrimination practices 28–9, 40, 150
Area Child Protection Committees 30, 32, 40, 80
area review committees 7
assessment 143
at risk 37
attachment 118
Auckland, Susan 10

Barnado's 101, 139
barrister 99
battered baby syndrome 10, 21
battered child
  research unit 6
  syndrome 5, 6
Beckford, Jasmine 11
behavioural
  characteristics of abuse 132
  indicators 77
  indicators of bullying 56
bonding 105, 106, 118
Bowlby, John 105, 106
bullying 55

Caffey 4
Camps, Dr 5
care order 31, 40
Carlile, Kimberley 11
challenging behaviour 154
characteristic behaviour 143
Cheshire 15
child abuse 60
  definition 42, 43
  inquiries 10, 15
child
  actors and models 17
  advocacy centres 40, 143
  assessment order 30, 40
  employment 16, 52, 60
  prostitution 51, 58, 60

child protection
  conference 7, 35, 36, 37, 86, 90
  orders 30
  plan 37, 90, 152
  register 6, 7, 37, 38, 58, 90
  register criteria 8
child psychiatrists 36, 94
child-care practitioner
  attending child protection conferences 36, 86, 125
  dealing with stress 129
  feelings when working with abused children 128
  giving evidence in court 126
  helping parents to understand abuse 145
  registration 39
  role 102
  role in preventing abuse 133
  as a role model 148
  the smacking debate 117
  supporting children in the criminal court 140
  working with abused children 135, 136
  working with parents who have abused 150
Childline 8, 11, 34, 58, 76, 101, 125
childminders 79
Children Act, 1989 9, 25, 26–7, 30, 85, 95, 125, 145, 147
Children's Society 101
children who abuse children 57
children with disabilities 138, 143
Children's legal centre 101
children's rights 22, 23, 24
Cleveland 8, 10, 12, 13, 21
Clwyd 15
Colwell, Maria 6, 10, 124
communicating
  with children 82, 120
  with colleagues 124
communication 130
confidentiality 125, 130
coping strategies 130
court clerk, 99
cultural differences 118